M000015180

Half Full

Half Full

Forty Inspiring Stories of Optimism, Hope, and Faith

Azriela Jaffe

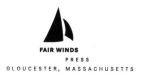

FAIR WINDS
PRESS
GLOUCESTER, MASSACHUSETTS

First published in the U.S.A. by
Fair Winds Press
33 Commercial Street
Gloucester, Massachusetts 01930-5089

Library of Congress Cataloging-in-Publication Data available

10 9 8 7 6 5 4 3 2 1

ISBN 1-931412-36-7

Cover design by Blue Anchor Design
Cover image by Getty Images
Design by Jill Feron/Feron Design

Printed and bound in Canada

This book is dedicated to my children, Sarah, Elana, and Elijah. Whenever something difficult occurs in my life, I have always been able to shift into a "half-full" attitude when I recognize how God has blessed me with three incredible, beautiful, healthy, smart children who love their mama and let her know that every day. With them as my greatest blessings, my life will never be anything but *totally* full.

Contents

Introduction

*I*t was smack in the middle of the dot-com craze. I was approached by a start-up firm run by a bunch of people with tight abs, hair that didn't need dye jobs, and unlimited energy that made 1:00 A.M. business meetings seem normal. They wanted me! The contract promised great wealth, the job description was right up my alley, and I could work from home four days a week. It seemed heaven-sent. My ship had finally come in.

And then, the ship sank, so swiftly, it seemed as if all those emails and meetings about my new job had been nothing but a dream. The stock market crashed, investors pulled out of any kind of dot-com start-up, and this company with multimillion-dollar potential evaporated into thin air. The twenty-somethings got other jobs or started some other entrepreneurial dream, and I returned to what I do best—writing books and my newspaper column.

I'd be lying to you if I said I never felt a moment of regret or mourning. The money would have been great. The job could have been fun. It felt really good for a few months to be pursued as a hot commodity. But honestly, I probably had a good pity-party for myself for a half a day, a day at most, and then I was back in full gear at my computer. Why? Because I live the principles of this book!

I immediately viewed the fiasco as good news in disguise. I didn't know why at that point. But I trusted that the universe had better plans for me. Maybe I would have gotten mugged in the subways of New York City. Perhaps I was born to write books, and getting caught up in a dot-com start-up would have diverted me from my true mission in life. Possibly I would have hated the job but felt trapped by my contract and the allure of so much money. Maybe one of my kids was going to need my attention in the future, and being involved in this job wouldn't have given me the flexibility I needed. I didn't know. It didn't really matter. When the opportunity disappeared, I maintained a "half-full" attitude. I decided, in the absence of any real data, to believe that this outcome was for the best.

When Paula Munier, acquiring editor for Fair Winds Press, the publisher of this book, approached me and asked me to write and edit this book for her, it was a no-brainer. She knew that I am the poster child for "half full" as a way of life. She was my editor at Adams Media, where we worked together on my book *Create Your Own Luck: Eight Principles of Attracting Good Fortune into Your Life, Love, and Work*, so she knew that I believed in creating your own reality with a positive attitude. She was also my editor on the *Heartwarmers* series, also published through Adams Media, a collection of true, heartwarming stories from authors all over the world. *Half Full* would be the perfect marriage of these two books: a book of true stories that illustrate looking at a challenge through "half full" eyes rather than "half-empty" ones.

I dove into this project with relish, and it scarcely felt like work. Subscribers to my free weekly newsletter, *Create Your Own Luck*, sent me their "half full" stories. Word circulated over the Internet, and some of my favorite *Heartwarmers* authors, and several new authors whom I did not know, sent me their stories for consideration. I wish we could have used them all.

You picked up this book because you too believe in maintaining an optimistic attitude about whatever challenge life throws your way. And, if you are like me, even though you are already convinced that a positive attitude is always within your reach, you love getting reminded. Read any one of the stories in this book, and you will feel more capable of handling whatever stress is in your life at this moment and more grateful that you don't have someone else's challenges. Read several of the stories, and you will understand that life is not enjoyed in spite of the problems we endure. Life is enjoyed because we have faced our challenges head-on, with an attitude of gratitude and a constant belief that whatever is happening in our lives is for the best.

Is your life half full or half empty? Only you can decide. Let the stories in this book inspire you to choose the half-full way of life.

"An Answered Prayer"

Deborah Dee Simmons

I implored the Lord, one tearful night,
to send me ideal days,
To grant me all my wishes, to smoothly
pave my way.
I pleaded for perfection, for months
without a care ...
An endless span of freedom from the
pain I could not bear.
I longed for warmth and sunshine, with
cloudless skies above,
And prayed for joy and laughter—and
never-ending love.
I craved respite from sorrow, from worries
and from strain,
I begged for peace and quiet—and
sought relief from pain.

But prayers for endless sunshine brought days of clouds and rain,

And pleas for sweet serenity bore times of stress and strain.

My petition for perfection brought me woes too great to bear ...

And desire for all my wishes—brought just worries and despair.

Despondent, tired, and burdened, I perused my dire plight,

And wondered why the Lord would seek to hinder what seemed right ...

For didn't I deserve release? So why was I denied?

Didn't He observe my pain—or hear my plaintive cry?

Couldn't God fulfill my wishes—and grant my every dream?

Just the smallest little miracle was all I'd need, it seemed ...

For my life to reach perfection—and my days to be sublime ...

Perhaps the Lord would hear me if I asked Him one more time.

So, again I fell upon my knees and prayed to God above,

But this time offered gratitude for His unending love.

I thanked Him for His bounty and the blessings He has wrought,

And miracles throughout my life I know His love has brought.

And soon, I found that happiness did far outweigh my woe,

As I sought the good in others—and reaped the seeds I sowed ...

I reveled in my blessings and the sweetness of my life,

And marveled at the strength I gained from dealing with my strife.

And yes, my prayers were answered—my appeals were not unheard,

I know that God has granted me the life that I deserve.

The miracle lay not in pleas—to free me from my strife ...

The miracle lay deep within—in how I viewed my life.

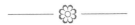

Deborah Simmons credits any past or future successes to God, Whose blessings include the inspiration He grants her whenever she sits down to write. To loosely quote Mark Twain, "God does the writing; I just take dictation." Since she's figured out that how we view our lives determines the good we are able to derive from it, Deb's found an endless supply of blessings and miracles to be grateful for each day. And speaking of blessings, Deb and her husband, John, live in mid-Michigan, relatively close to their two sons, their wives, and three of their grandchildren. Their youngest daughter and her husband, who is in the army, and their baby son live in Tennessee. Their oldest daughter and her husband, who serves in the air force, live on the Eielson Air Force Base just south of Fairbanks, Alaska.

Serendipity

Risë Kittle

*S*erendipity! I've always liked that word, the finding of something so special or treasured when least expected. While it's not a word I use every day, it describes what happened to my life in January 2001.

I had finally found a full-time job that would allow me to put the youngest of my four boys on the school bus each morning. Life was better to my two younger boys and me than it had been for quite some time. I was a single mom, and we knew that sacrifices were to be expected. My son, Jared (fourteen), would get his brother, Zachary (eight), off the bus, feed him supper, help with homework, get him ready for bed, and read him a story. Child support was very sporadic, so we worked together to stay off welfare and keep our house. My two older sons, Jeremy (twenty-three) and John (twenty-one), would stop by as their schedules allowed. My new job started January 15.

On January 12, a young mother shot and killed her husband and then herself. I did not know them personally. However, the young mother's cousin by marriage was given custody of her four daughters. That cousin, Shannon, is very special to me, as she married one of Jeremy's best friends, Brady. She is actually like a daughter to me. Having had four brothers and no sisters and then four boys and no girls of my own, it is indeed a treasure here to have another female around!

Shannon called me the evening of the twelfth to ask me if I had heard about the murder-suicide approximately twenty miles from my home and to inform me that the police had allowed her to take the four orphans to her home. I told her to keep me updated as to how things were going. Throughout the following two weeks, she and I continued to call each other. On January 28, Shannon and Brady brought the oldest girl, Alia, to visit me. They were feeling quite overwhelmed with the responsibility of their own little boy and all the girls. The girls were divided and sleeping with different relatives, and then spending all day with Shannon. Even though I was working five and a half days a week, I offered to take all the children from a Saturday afternoon until either Sunday night or Monday morning. My lifelong dream of having little girls around had been reawakened!

I'd never met the family, but I wasn't worried, since before taking a full-time office job, for five years I was a foster mom to twenty-four children. I wasn't overly concerned about how we'd manage, because I've had abused children removed from terrible conditions in big cities and brought directly to me with no background information. My prayer was that if this was meant to be that God would give me a sign, either by closing doors or showing me beyond any doubt that I was capable of handling the situation.

After work the following Saturday, the four girls came. This was the first night that they had all spent together since the tragedy. I wasn't mentally prepared to see the terrible physical condition of the children. The two youngest had thick cradle cap and blisters on their bottoms from not having their diapers changed. Angel was thirty-three months old, and not potty trained. All four girls were so congested they couldn't breathe through their noses. The two littlest had been staying with a family member that had twenty cats in the house and they reeked of cat pee. The children were malnourished and developmentally delayed. The baby cried and cried, and I just held her and rocked her most of the night.

Something happened in my heart that night as I held this poor innocent child in my arms, knowing she needed to be loved and cared for. There had to be a reason they had been brought into my life. When Shannon had placed the baby in my arms and said, "Here's your daughter, Mom!" I really didn't know if I could do the job of loving and protecting them, but I worried that after all the girls had been through, they would be divided into different homes if they were put into foster care or adopted.

Throughout the night, as we rocked, I was haunted by the painful memory of how, in a breaking point after years of an abusive marriage and the devastating loss of my mother, I had put a loaded pistol to my head. Had it not been for my indecision of whether to put the bullet through my mouth or the right side of my head, and the quick action of one of God's angels, I would have left my own four boys to be divided among family members. My pastor "just happened" to stop by at that time to tell us about the Vacation Bible School, and I sobbed as I poured my heart out to him about the deep hurt I couldn't make go away.

It took many months of focusing on the positive things in my life, counseling, and the support of my very dear friends for me to put my life back together. I almost left four boys to be orphaned, like these girls were. I hurt for the little girls' mom who didn't feel she had any other option or friends to turn to for help.

By morning I knew what I had to do.

The next day, the step-grandmother and Shannon's mother came to pick the girls up so I could go back to work. Alia, ten years old, walked quietly to the car; she had made up her mind that she wanted to come back to my home. Jared carried Stariel, five years old, out to the car, and she cried. Angel clung to my neck as I promised her I'd see her the next weekend. The baby, Rhiannon, seventeen months old, sat in the car seat and just looked at me as if to say, "Why do I have to go?" My arms felt as empty as the look in their eyes. As they pulled out of our driveway, Jared looked at me and said, "Mom, you know that you have to fight to keep them together."

When I returned to work, I gave my notice to a very surprised supervisor. He told me he hoped it worked out, and that if I wanted my job back, it would be waiting for me. That week the family members offered to give me Alia and Angel. But I didn't want the children to be split up. The step-grandmother offered to keep the baby but planned to put her into day care, since she worked. I asked her to let me have the children throughout the week and then take them together on the weekends.

Brady had developed a real bond with Alia and wanted a chance to work with her, to allow her to be a child and not have the responsibility of raising her three younger half sisters. Alia had never received her immunizations, been to school, or known what it was like to settle into a real family life. Her mother and stepfather had been to forty-two states in five years, living off the Social Security Survivor Death Benefits from Alia's father, who had passed away in 1992. Alia was the most in need of extra attention, since she was the one who had discovered the bodies and had closed her stepdaddy's eyes.

Children and Youth services made the decision they felt was in the best interest of the children. The judge gave me, a single parent, temporary legal custody, with the supervision of Children and Youth, of the three little girls. Alia would stay with Shannon and Brady. When I asked about becoming an active foster parent again and was informed that the children would then become eligible for separate adoption after a year, I opted to use welfare benefits to make ends meet.

People tell me they think I'm wonderful for taking on the responsibility of someone else's children. I feel as though I am the one who is blessed. I had a hysterectomy and then received three more children! My boys have bonded so well with my girls that it's hard for any of us to remember when they weren't here.

We've worked hard for more than a year now. The girls had never had an immunization shot. I cried as much as they did when I held each one as they were given sixteen shots apiece! Stariel had to have nine cavities filled, and Angel three. Stariel started school and does very well. Night after night I've sat with her doing homework, erasing backward letters and numbers, wondering how she felt about having to struggle so hard to catch up to her peers. One night she commented "Mommy, I love you! Do you know how special it is to have someone to teach me how to do my homework right?" The tears ran down my face as I responded, "Do you know how special you are and how happy I am that you are here with me?"

Angel potty-trained for me within the first two weeks of being here. She called me Risë until the other children asked her, "Why don't you ever call her Mommy?" She responded, "My real mommy died, so she is only my fake mommy!" We all laughed, but ever since then, she is the most insistent that I be called "Mommy."

Rhiannon potty-trained for me at twenty-six months. She sings, dances, says her ABC's, and counts to ninety-nine with a little help. She has long, dark hair like mine, and complete strangers comment on how much my daughter looks like me. At times she calls me "Mommy Daddy" to the delight of all who know us. She sings "You Are My Sunshine," and indeed, she is ours.

In July, the intake worker from Children and Youth petitioned the court to give me full legal custody and for them to be dropped from the case. Normally, they would have been involved for a minimum of two years, but when the caseworker saw the kids in January, she couldn't believe they were the same children. She was amazed with how much we have bonded and with their progress: physical, social, emotional, and academic.

In October, the judge simply asked me if I wanted to keep the little girls forever. I tearfully responded, "Oh, yes, I've waited all my life for them!"

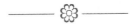

By the time this story is published, Risë and her entire family will have relocated to property left to her children by her first husband. They will be living in Georgia, on two and a half acres of land with a small trailer they can live in, while they build a new life in a new area of the country. She and her children are very excited about a new start in life. They are confident that as long as they are together, with God's continued blessings, they will survive any hardships that come their way.

Sometimes You Don't Know the Reason Why ...

Anonymous

The only survivor of a shipwreck was washed up on a small, uninhabited island. He prayed feverishly for God to rescue him, and every day he scanned the horizon for help, but none seemed forthcoming. Exhausted, he eventually managed to build a little hut out of driftwood to protect him from the elements and to store his few possessions.

But then one day, after scavenging for food, he arrived home to find his little hut in flames, the smoke rolling up to the sky. The worst had happened; everything was lost. He was stunned with grief and anger.

"God, how could you do this to me?" he cried.

Early the next day, however, he was awakened by the sound of a ship approaching the island. It had come to rescue him.

"How did you know I was here?" asked the weary man of his rescuers.

"We saw your smoke signal," they replied.

It is easy to get discouraged when things are going bad. But we shouldn't lose heart, because God is at work in our lives, even in the midst of pain and suffering. Remember, next time your little hut is burning to the ground it just may be a smoke signal that summons the grace of God.

Monkey Bars

Sally Friedman

I am, by nature, a pessimistic person. Always have been. But people do change, even in late middle age. My moment came on an outing with Jonah, our irrepressible firecracker of a four-year-old grandson.

We were heading for the playground, where Jonah is something of a daredevil and I am a confirmed coward. Jonah was already outlining for me what he'd do—his own version of the feats of Hercules. He would swing "higher than the sky" on the swings. He would do ten chin-ups on the bars. And he would climb to the tippy-top of the jungle gym.

I listened with a grandmother's pride. This kid was tough, determined, and brave: something I'd never be!

At each playground stop, Jonah lived up to his self-billing. He did swing higher than I imagined a four-year-old ever could. He managed those chin-ups, struggling by the end, but triumphant. And then we got to the jungle gym. As I stared up at it, a thousand images flashed before my eyes.

I was ten and the only kid in the playground who *knew* I couldn't handle that accursed piece of torturous equipment. I tried to hide my shame and to disappear behind the schoolyard wall, but Harvey, the class bully, spotted me. And he showed no mercy.

"Baby, baby! Stick your head in gravy!" was his chant. And as others joined in, I surrendered to the tears that I couldn't hold back.

All of this came flooding back as Jonah began his own climb. Surefooted and fast, he was a study in confidence. How I envied him. And then Jonah looked down at me, and I saw something in that face that I'd never seen before. It was a mix of sadness, sympathy, and frustration.

"C'mon, Grandma," he urged. "You can do it."

No way! I was now sixty years old. I surely wasn't going to attempt something I couldn't even manage when I was ten and, theoretically, agile.

Jonah kept at it, with that persistence only four-year-olds can muster.

"Grandma," he finally said, "just tell your brain that you can!"

It was one of those moments. That simple instruction from a four-year-old penetrated something deep, deep in my psyche. "Tell your brain that you can!"

I took a deep breath and put one sneakered foot on the lowest bar. I made it to the next and almost bolted. But

Jonah was just above me, his eyes dancing with delight, my silent cheerleader.

I got to the next level, and the next.

And suddenly, astoundingly, I was on the top of those monkey bars, feeling like I'd just climbed Everest.

And maybe I had.

Jonah seemed to sense that this was more than just a clumsy grandma acting like a kid. "You *did* it!" he beamed. "You *did* it, Grandma."

And suddenly it didn't matter that eons ago, I'd been the target of the playground meanies. It didn't matter that Harvey had aimed those childhood slings and arrows right through my heart and my pride. What mattered was that I'd tasted optimism—and it was delicious.

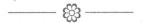

Sally is a graduate of the University of Pennsylvania, an English major who fell in love with words as a kid. She has been a freelance writer and columnist for thirty years and contributes to regional and national publications. Her work has appeared in the *New York Times*, the *Philadelphia Inquirer*, *Ladies' Home Journal*, *Family Circle*, and *Bride's*, among other publications.

Her best work has been three daughters, five grandchildren, and a wonderful marriage to Victor, a retired New Jersey superior court judge.

Sweet Sarah

Azriela Jaffe

When I married my husband, Stephen, I was thirty-four, and my biological clock had been ticking loudly for a few years. I didn't want to wind up pregnant at forty.

We hoped for a nice sentimental story—pregnant on the honeymoon, and our first child within a year. God delivered. I was pregnant before we returned from our honeymoon, according to the home pregnancy test I took a few weeks later. We were elated. It felt like an affirmation of our love for one another, the rightness of our union, and a dream come true.

I was terribly ill for the first two months of the pregnancy, throwing up every day, often several times a day, and losing almost ten pounds, which I really didn't have to lose. Stephen marveled at my ability to wake up, vomit, and then get on with my day, as if it were no big deal. It wasn't fun, but I was so grateful to be pregnant that I took it in stride.

One evening, about ten weeks into the pregnancy, I lay in bed feeling particularly miserable. My stomach hurt worse than usual, more like menstrual cramping than nausea. I rose to go to the bathroom and was horrified to discover that I was bleeding. We contacted our midwife, and she gave me instructions. It wasn't long before the truth was revealed: I had miscarried.

Any woman who has ever experienced this fate, and so many of us have, knows the grief that washes over you at this moment. It was one of the worst losses of my life. I was losing not only a life growing inside of me, but also a dream. I was terrified—did this mean that I would have difficulty conceiving or carrying a baby to term? I mourned for the little girl, or boy, whom we had lost.

Sarah Jaffe, sweet Sarah, our oldest daughter, age eight now, was conceived a few months later. If I had known at the time that God had such an incredible gift in store for us, I would have accepted the miscarriage with greater ease. If I had known what I know now, by being her mother, I would have still mourned the miscarriage, but I would have recovered more quickly from it. Only in hindsight was I able to have complete faith that it was meant to be, and in the context of my life, understand that the miscarriage was a positive, not a negative event.

Every mother loves her daughter. Every mother will tell you that her daughter is one of the finest human beings ever to be born.

But really, Sarah is.

The daycare staff labeled her "easy money" because she was always such a joy to be around. She wakes up happy, she giggles throughout the day, and she spends many of her waking moments trying to figure out how to be kind to others. She is so stunningly beautiful that complete strangers walk up to me and tell me that I had better watch out when she becomes a teenager. She is the child who gave up her favorite "blanky" to keep someone warm and will come up to her tired mother and say, "Mama, you work too hard. Is there anything I can do for you today?"

One of my favorite memories of Sarah goes back to my second pregnancy with her sister, Elana, when I was so ill, parked on the couch and waiting for waves of nausea to dissipate. Sarah was concerned, and so she lay down next to me and extended her sucking thumb, saying, "Suck this, Mama, it always makes me feel better, and it will make you feel better too!"

When Sarah announces to me, "Mama, I love you bigger than God," I never get tired of hearing it. I could not possibly feel more love for a human being than I feel for my daughter Sarah.

I never forget that Sarah was born only because I miscarried. In God's great plan, not mine, the baby before Sarah was not meant to be in our family. Sarah definitely was. Sarah reminds me every day that God's plan is usually better than my own. When life isn't going the way I had planned, I think of my sweet Sarah, and I await the blessings that God has in store for me.

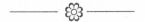

Azriela didn't have to worry about her biological clock running out after all. She gave birth to three healthy babies in four years—Sarah, Elana, and Elijah, before she hit her fortieth birthday. Azriela published three books during that time, so everyone wondered: Could she write a fourth book without producing a fourth child? Did she have to be pregnant to write a book? She's delighted to say that she's now the author of twelve books, but her biological children remain at three.

Standing Up for Downhill

Gene Ledue

"How's your courage?" my supervisor, Jim, asked me. In my years as a volunteer ski instructor at Maine Handicapped Skiing the question had never been posed to me.

I'm an avid skier, grateful that I am still walking. I once skied off a trail going much too fast and after two somersaults and many missed trees, I landed on my back on two large snowmaking pipes about thirty feet down in a gully.

It took me about an hour to climb back up those thirty feet, since my back kept spasming. The ski patrol marveled that if I were not so thickly muscled I would have suffered a much worse fate. I suffered only deep bruising on my back and legs.

Not too long afterward, I saw an ad in a local periodical placed by someone looking for volunteer ski instructors for the physically disabled. Realizing how lucky I was, I knew it was time to give something back to those who were not as fortunate as I am. Over the past thirteen years as a volunteer, I have received more in return than I could have imagined. Many, many skiers have touched my heart.

One woman taught me about courage. Jen, my teaching challenge of the day, was a bright, pretty woman in her twenties with strawberry-blond hair and a comfortable manner. Yet something was unnerving me.

It wasn't her disability. Jen suffered an injury to her neck as a result of a hit-and-run accident that occurred when she was thirteen. Jen is a quadriplegic who struggles to keep weight on, no small physical challenge but not one that was unusual for the MHS program. MHS opens its doors to the whole spectrum of people with their different disabilities.

It wasn't Jen's attitude. Jen possesses unbridled enthusiasm and optimism. She has a good sense of humor, is terrifically confident, and never squanders a moment feeling dismayed or looking at limits. This is inspiring stuff, but MHS is a magnet for people with these attributes. I think back to my first student, Samuel, a five-year-old with spina bifida. In exchange for taking him on his first chairlift ride and guiding his discovery of skiing, he warmed my heart, wiped my sweaty brow, and gave me that special feeling that comes with being someone's hero. I keep coming back because of people like Jen and Samuel. But no, they're not unusual for MHS.

Jen's reason for coming to MHS was not unusual either. She spends most of her day in a wheelchair. Like us, she was drawn to do the downhill dance for the feeling of the wind and sun in her face and the freedom and exhilaration of gliding on a carpet of snow crystals.

What was unusual and what was unnerving me was Jen's desire and determination to ski standing up. Because of the severity of her spinal cord injury, her doctors said it couldn't be done. In fact, it had never been attempted. I fought my impulse to recommend a BI-SKI, an adaptive piece of ski equipment that would allow Jen to experience greater skiing success sooner, but from a sitting position.

Jen had her own vision and was undaunted. She set out to prove her doctors (and, unknowingly, me) wrong. Jen brought along a new and innovative full-body brace that enabled her to sustain a standing position. Together with my MHS cohorts, I sought a way to adapt ski equipment that allowed her to ski in an upright position.

This was new territory, virtually untracked powder from the skiing perspective. Paula, the executive director of MHS, noticed us collaborating on one of our initial creations for Jen. "Ah, the art of adaptive skiing!" Paula exclaimed. In MHS's thirteen-year history, Paula has seen many solutions materialize; once again we would find a way.

Our final concoction for Jen included the following ingredients: a walker with skis attached to the bottom, skis for Jen with tips kept together by a ski bra, a bamboo pole across the front of the walker to enable instructors to assist, and bungee cords to keep ski equipment and skier in sync. To this we added courage, enthusiasm, teamwork, and some snow and gravity. Incredibly, before the day was done, Jen was skiing upright and loving it.

Photographs were taken for her doctors and for posterity, but her ski adventure had just begun. Before the season was over Jen was cruising down the mountain with a little help from her friends at MHS. There were hurdles to clear along the way and the occasional showstopper, but we could always count on Jen's positive outlook. In her upbeat way, she supported us when there was a setback, saying, "That's okay! We did great today, and we can do even better next week!"

She taught me to hold on to my dreams and to respect the dreams of others, to see the possibilities and set no limits, to feel the fear and do it anyway. Ultimately she gave me an answer to a question that would come up again: *How's your courage?*

Gene first volunteered at Maine Handicapped Skiing in 1989. In 2002, the twentieth anniversary year of MHS, Gene continued his involvement as a volunteer instructor and captain of a fund-raising team for the MHS skiathon. The skiathon is a one-day event that raises 95 percent of the funding for this free program. Gene lives in South Portland, Maine, with his wife, Teri, and their three children, Emily, James, and Olivia.

From Bars to Books

Bill Asenjo

*M*y journey to getting a Ph.D. and becoming a published writer began in 1985 with a brain tumor. At the time I was a thirty-six-year-old card-carrying Peter Pan, thinly disguised as a hard-drinking, unemployed bartender. Responsibility was not my strong suit.

The tumor introduced itself during a poker game, blinding and paralyzing me. Without warning, the lights went out, and I plopped facedown on the table like a puppet with its strings cut. With my face pressed against the cool, hard Formica table, I thought I was dying. Not the way I pictured the end.

It wasn't the end. So much for the good news. The bad news, the doctors announced, was that I had a brain tumor. "Bigger than a golf ball," is how the neurosurgeon described it.

They opened me up in surgery to see what they'd find. There were complications. After six months in the hospital, six surgeries, spinal meningitis, and several close calls, I emerged damaged, shaken, but alive. Because the tumor had been so difficult to remove, the surgeons recommended periodic testing to make sure the stubborn, but thankfully noncancerous, tumor had not grown back. As I was told, once you have a brain tumor you're more likely to have another one.

My next step on the journey was a rehab program and counseling. Perhaps I should have been grateful to be alive, but frankly, my attitude was terrible. My mantra? "Poor me." A no-nonsense counselor responded to my version of thumb sucking by saying, "Sympathy's in the dictionary, Bill, between sweat and syphilis." He knew I needed an attitude adjustment—fast—so he recommended that I help others with disabilities to help me stop drowning in self-pity.

Grumbling the whole way, I did what he told me. After reading for a man who had lost his sight and working with children in wheelchairs, I was surprised to find that I was enjoying myself. It was nearly impossible to suck my thumb while offering that same hand in help to someone else.

After a year or so, I recovered sufficiently to get on with my life. My sister summed it up nicely. "Let's see," she said one day as we discussed my future, "you're disabled, you flunked out of college, and you have no marketable skills." We both pondered that résumé. "Maybe you should register for some classes at the junior college. See how you do."

Not sure what else to do, I found myself waiting to register, while wondering if I was too damaged or—at nearly thirty-eight years old—too old, to do something with my life. I got in, of course: junior colleges admit anybody with a pulse.

Returning to a classroom was surreal. Surrounded by seventeen-year-olds, I felt like Michael J. Fox in *Back to the Future*. Although several of my permanent disabilities were invisible, such as deafness in one ear and damaged vision, the surgeries also caused some brain damage that interfered with my balance. As a result, I often lost my balance even when standing still. And my appearance attracted some attention. Part of my skull had not been replaced behind my left ear, which could only be partially disguised by letting my hair grow long, and the end of a very thick Frankenstein scar was still plainly visible on the back of my neck.

My impaired vision was perhaps my most troublesome disability. Other parts of the printed page would superimpose on the text I was trying to read. Until I adjusted my eyes, it took forever to read anything, and, of course, it led to some interesting misinterpretations.

That first semester I worried about passing. Grades were posted, and I saw my name—with straight A's next to it. I thought it was my vision. I did a double take so fast I could have pulled a muscle in my neck. After the registrar's office assured me the grades were accurate, I was thrilled.

After four years I received a bachelor's degree, and because I tried several graduate programs it took me another four years to earn my master's in health science, specializing in rehabilitation counseling. In 2001 I completed my Ph.D. dissertation on alternative medical therapies for people with disabilities. That year I also received the $2,500 grand prize for the best-written dissertation at the Fifteenth International Conference on Human Functioning. Along the way I chameleoned into a freelance writer, a profession I didn't even know I had always wanted.

I've been fortunate to have a second chance at life. In an effort to repay what I consider a debt of gratitude, I spend much of my spare time helping people with disabilities. As a result, today my life has purpose and meaning, something I always wanted but never knew how to find.

I'd probably still be tending bar. If it weren't for that brain tumor.

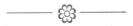

Bill Asenjo, Ph.D., is a freelance writer, college instructor, certified rehabilitation counselor (C.R.C.), and healthcare consultant. In a former lifetime—before multiple brain tumor surgeries—Bill had been a bartender, New York City cab driver, college dropout, construction worker, and truck driver, among other less-illustrious occupations.

I Am the One

Carol A. Meyer

I inherited a legacy of negativity and pain, especially from my family on my father's side. My grandparents divorced when my father was young, and there was almost nothing said regarding my grandfather that was positive. In fact, there was almost nothing said at all. My father never spoke about my grandfather with my mother, and since I was two and a half when my father died, I was unable to ask him directly about my grandfather. My grandmother also refused to speak of him, although she was the one who sent me the clipping from the newspaper about his death, with no comment. I became determined to find his gravesite and to put closure to this painful legacy.

Many years ago, my husband and I planned a weekend away with friends to look at the general area where my grandfather had lived—Poughkeepsie, New York. We did some research by calling funeral homes in the area and asking about the local cemeteries. It was unfruitful; no one could tell me where my grandfather was buried.

In the summer of 2000, I was drawn back to school after a long hiatus to earn my master's in transpersonal studies. I was fortunate to have Angeles Arrien, the author of *The Four-Fold Way*, present at the opening seminar of my first year. One of her points kept reverberating through my mind. She wanted us to know that earlier generations stand behind us to help us through our lives, and they ask, "Will you be the one?"

What this question meant was, Will you be the one to break the negative patterns that can endure in a family for generations. In the fall of 2000 I took a course titled "A Transpersonal Approach to Family Systems" that gave me an opportunity to search for patterns in my family history through the generations? As I read the books that accompanied the course, I kept hearing Angeles Arrien's words at that opening class. I decided that I would be "the one."

My course paper became a letter to specific family groups addressing what I had learned about their impact on my life. After much interviewing the few family members alive that would possibly know anything, I decided to try to get any military records and a death certificate for my paternal grandfather. It was a needle-in-a-haystack struggle, since the "facts" about my grandfather were precious few, other than the date of death and the name of the town where he died.

After a few false starts and encounters with some helpful people, I sent money and request forms to the addresses that I felt were the most likely sources. Within a month I held a copy of my grandfather's death certificate in my hands. I had a lot more facts now, including where he was buried. I called the town clerk of Highland Falls, New York, where the Peace Dale cemetery is located and was given a name of a gentleman that "knew everything about everybody in town."

When I had a copy of my grandfather's military discharge information in hand, my husband and I made plans to search for his gravesite while we were vacationing in the Pocono Mountains, even though it was a detour of several hours.

On Sunday morning, May 26, 2002, we arrived in the town around noon. As we drove down the main street I suddenly saw one of those "you are here" signs. What luck, the sign pointed the way to the cemetery! We ate lunch in a Mexican restaurant before going to the cemetery, appropriate since my grandfather had served in the Spanish-American War. After lunch, we drove into the cemetery, which was peaceful and absolutely beautiful. There was only one other car there, and as we drove near I told my husband to let me out so that I could ask questions of the driver. She was very friendly and by a stroke of luck turned out to be the town clerk. She shared that there had been vandalism at the cemetery after the flags had been placed on the graves in preparation for the Memorial Day weekend, so I could not count on a flag as a clue.

We had approximately two square city blocks to cover. We were walking at the base of the lovely rock outcropping about one hundred yards from the road when my husband said, "There it is!" What luck—it only took five minutes to locate the grave among all the others in the cemetery.

Just like that, fifty-eight years of separation came to an end. As I turned to look my heartbeat quickened. I gazed at my grandfather's grave and thought with some sadness of the missed opportunities in our lives. The gravestone was larger than I had expected and showed signs of weather and the ground sinking away from it. It was standing proudly upright showing a cross inscribed within a circle, his name, New York PVT (Private) USMA (United States Military Academy) DET (Detached) CAV (Cavalry), and his birth and death dates. I checked my information, and everything matched. The flag holder was at the side of the grave where the vandals had thrown it, and with determination I picked it up and pushed it into the ground next to the stone.

I silently spoke to my grandmother, father, and uncle. I asked that they forgive this man for the pain he had caused them. My search for his gravesite was the manifestation of a longing for a sense of connection, a feeling of completion, and a way to honor my paternal heritage. No one is perfect, and everyone has gifts to bring to this world. One of my grandfather's gifts to me was to have me understand just how influential my decisions in life will be on future generations. Because of my grandfather's legacy, I will work harder to heal the pain that previous generations have willed to me. Hopefully, I will leave a much different legacy to my children and grandchildren. I am definitely "the one."

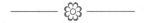

Carol is certified as a handwriting consultant. She expects to earn her master's in transpersonal studies from the Institute of Transpersonal Psychology in Palo Alto, California, and also to become a certified teacher of the Enneagram. Carol honors all who have taught her to love herself and others—most especially her husband and their three sons. Carol and her husband were thrilled to learn, only eleven days after returning from her grandfather's gravesite, that they are going to be grandparents for the first time.

Home, Sweet Home

Cheryl Russell

*I*always wanted to own a home of my own. But not just any home. No, I had a very particular, and some would say, peculiar, idea of what my home would look like. Just about everyone in my life said it was "impossible." But impossible is all in the mind. I never gave up on my dream, and now I've got an amazing house to show for it.

In 1998, when I first took a job for the local La Crosse Area Realtors Association in La Crosse, Wisconsin, one of my duties was cataloging and processing photos of newly listed properties. I'd often look at a photo and muse about the features I did or did not like. This led me to be able to visualize what type of house I would someday buy for my family.

After two years, I decided to start looking more closely at the prospects for buying a house. I had a fairly extensive list of wants:

- two-story home with at least 1,800 square feet of space
- at least a half-acre of land
- three or more good-sized bedrooms
- formal dining room and large kitchen
- cathedral ceilings
- nice woodwork and detail: character
- lots of closet or storage space
- wood or tile floors throughout
- more than one bathroom
- all this for less than $75,000

I mentioned my interest in purchasing a home to several realtors I knew through my work, but once they saw my list of wants and heard what I was willing to pay, they scoffed, telling me I'd never find such a house for that price. While it was discouraging, I kept talking to agents until I found one who was willing to attempt to help me find the house we wanted.

I entered into a buyer agency agreement with a realtor, but I was disappointed in most of the homes she showed me; they were small, one-story bungalows and ranch homes with few, if any, of the features on my list. She thought I was deranged in thinking my ideals could be had for my desired price!

I wouldn't give up, however. I found financing in a program designed for low- to middle-income families. We continued to look, and I remained optimistic, despite the odds. The realtor finally showed me a small home that, despite being ranch style, was somewhat charming. It had a one-acre plot, which afforded plenty of room for building an addition. I felt that there was potential there, so we agreed to write an offer. The offer was accepted, the financing was in place, and the closing date was tentatively set, pending the home inspection. On the date of the inspection, I was ready to make an emotional commitment to this home. I had peace. It would work.

Or not. The home inspection revealed damage to the west wall of the foundation. Some of the concrete bricks were not original. The current owners vehemently denied that information and refused to hire an engineer to verify if the home's foundation was secure. Without an engineer's approval, my lender would not proceed with the loan. The house of my dreams was not this one.

The following spring, my family and I had yet to give up hope. We decided to drive around some of the surrounding towns to see what had come on the market. To our amazement, we saw that a small gambrel-roofed home with a view of the Mississippi River that had been for sale the previous fall was once again on the market!

Even though the house was a bit on the small side, it did have the potential for a nice addition to the front that would almost double its size. If the price was right, we thought, we might consider it. We peeked in the windows and found the front porch to be unlocked. Going in, we found a large window opening to the main floor. The house felt open. There was wood galore, and character. I was salivating. This is the house I wanted!

With the pre-approval process in place, and a new realtor, Katy, we set up a showing. We made an offer instantaneously. The seller accepted our offer readily, and we set up appointments for the inspections and appraisal. Everything was going well, so I gave our landlord a thirty-day notice. The house was vacant, so we could close and move in quickly!

Less than two weeks before the closing, I was packing furiously and trying to arrange all the details, like getting utilities hooked up, dealing with change of address notifications, and more. Katy called me, telling me that we might have a problem. The appraiser was having a hard time finding enough value in the house to meet the sale price. If he could not justify the sale price, the lender would not go through with the closing!

Two days later, the final appraisal report came in. It was nowhere near the sale price. The seller's agent told Katy not to even consider counteroffering to lower the sale price, because the seller simply would not do it. I was in shock. In fact, I was petrified. My landlord had informed me that he had new tenants ready to move in as soon as we could vacate. My family and I were to be homeless.

Somehow, I got past the momentary shock and decided that if this house was also not the right one for me, there must be a reason. There must be something else out there that we had missed. Katy scoured the listings of all the area agents, hoping to find something just right, just listed, and just-so-happened-to-be-available for a quick closing. Nothing.

The next day I was at work when a staff person at one of the real estate companies called me to check that an open house request that she had faxed had arrived. "It's very important that this open house take place," she said. "The sellers want it sold quickly!" I asked her for the address as I leafed through the pile of faxes.

When I found it, I assured her that it had been received and would be included in the directory that weekend. She thanked me and hung up, while I continued to glance at the information about the house. Hmm, in De Soto? Katy had searched the computer database for homes in De Soto and hadn't found this one. Hmm, price was right. Hmm, remodeled farmhouse, new siding, new furnace, new plumbing, open style, more than half an acre? This might be worth looking into!

I pounced on Katy as soon as she emerged from a meeting. "Katy! Look at this!"

She read the sheet, taking in the same information that had struck me. Vacant. Great price. Within minutes, we had flown out the door and were headed south to De Soto, feeling the vibes that this was what we had been waiting for. As we approached the middle of De Soto, we noticed a sign on the highway. It informed us that we were now entering Crawford County. Half the village is in Vernon County, and that's where Katy had searched in the computer. She had not located this house in her searching, because neither of us realized that the village was split by a county line!

When we pulled up to the house, the remnants of a late spring snowstorm were still on the walk, but the sun was shining and the white siding shone. We picked through the slush and Katy unlocked the door, sticking her head in the doorway. I tried vainly to see around her trademark cowboy hat but could not. She quickly pulled the door shut and turned around saying, "Nah, you're not gonna like this one."

The panic in my eyes made her laugh, and she swiftly assured me she was joking. She then swung the door open and we entered, our breaths taken away by the sight of the living room we were standing in. It had a cathedral ceiling ... with a loft, no less! Ten feet of built-in bookshelves surrounded the double doorway to the middle of the house. Hardwood floors, woodwork everywhere, and charm galore!

The afternoon sun from the south side of the house drew us through the double doorway, and turning left, we entered the largest, most amazing kitchen! Thirty feet of white cupboards lined two of the walls, with dark green ceramic tile on the floor and a patio door leading to a deck.

We each took off in different directions, yelling out our finds as we went along: "Katy, there's a bathroom here, off the kitchen!" "Cheryl, there's a bathroom here off the master bedroom!" "Katy, did you see the closets in this bedroom?" "Cheryl, you have *got* to come look at this bay window," and so on. Within five minutes, we had scrambled through the two-thousand-square-foot house, breathless with the wonder of every new discovery.

In all we found three huge bedrooms, three full baths, lots of closets in each room, the huge kitchen, the glorious living room with the loft, a formal dining room, yet another large room joining the dining room with yet another double doorway, and an unfinished three-season porch with a view of the Mississippi River!

We didn't stay long, so urgent were we in getting back to her office to write the offer. My heart sunk momentarily. What if an offer had already been accepted, or there had been a mistake in the posted price? Surely this home was worth way more than $75,000? Katy assured me that she'd send the offer to the listing company immediately and ask the sellers for a response within twenty-four hours, since we now only had ten days before we had to vacate our apartment. I felt that this house was to be ours!

Later that afternoon, Katy called to tell me that the listing company had received another offer on the house, just that afternoon, but it had not been faxed to the sellers yet, who lived in another state. So ours would be presented at the same time as the other offer. If the sellers had our full-price offer on the table, knowing that the closing could take place in ten days and they'd have their money, we would likely win the deal. I agreed, telling her, "Just get me that house!"

It was a long, agonizing wait through the next twenty-four hours until we heard back from the listing agent. The house was ours, for $73,500. Even in a village thirty miles away from the main city of La Crosse, it was a steal! The sellers (a minister and his wife) had been transferred out of state a few years earlier and they just wanted to break even and sell it fast.

I cried tears of triumph and relief. While I was always sure in my heart, it was a relief to have the actual signed acceptance papers in my hands. With very few snags, other than the terrible weather on moving day, the deal was settled, and we moved in. All in ten days.

I'll never forget how many friends, family members, and even real estate agents told me we'd never find this house at this price. I dreamed big, I believed, and even though I lost faith a few times and almost bought the wrong house, my optimism eventually paid off!

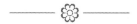

Cheryl and Fred have lived in the house for two years with her thirteen-year-old daughter, Sarah, their newborn baby, and a passel of pet birds, reptiles, and rodents. Every time she returns home, she still says to herself, "Wow! That's our house!" She hopes to be able to start a cottage industry in sewing so that eventually she can work from home while caring for her family.

The Last Kiss

Connie Feste Wooldridge

My husband, Jon, and I were poor college students when we moved into our second little apartment located directly across from the college tennis courts and parking lot. Both of us went to classes early in the day and worked at night. We only had one car, so that meant I had to pick him up at the factory warehouse after I got off work at a local pizza place. We argued if I was the least bit late, because then he would have someone take him home and I would show up at the factory and sit wondering where he could be. After arguing, I assured him that I would always pick him up and made him promise to wait until I got there.

On this particular day I got home early enough to turn on one of those wonderful old romantic movies. Soon it was time for Jon to get off work, but I had not seen the last kiss. I put on my shoes, coat, hat, and gloves. I picked up my keys and purse and inched backward through the front door as I watched the final minutes. Finally the leading man grabbed the girl and kissed her; I hurried out the door and took off toward the parking lot at a dead run, worried that my husband would be angry at me for keeping him waiting.

I felt myself slammed to the ground so quickly that I didn't even know what had happened. I felt the pavement hard against my cheek; my arm was twisted, and my glasses mangled. My purse was open and its contents scattered. My whole body ached. Had I been mugged?

Once I had my wits about me, I realized that I had run into a car parked along my street. It was so dark I had not seen it. I slammed into it with such force that I must have sailed like a cartoon character over the top of the hood and into the street.

My next thought was about that promise Jon had made to wait for me. I could not walk. Somehow I dragged myself back to the apartment and pulled myself up to the telephone. I dialed the number of the factory and asked to speak to my husband. "It's an emergency," I whimpered. When Jon came to the phone I began to cry and feebly managed to tell him I was home and had been in an accident. He got a ride home, and rushed into our home. He only had to take one look at me, and we were off to the emergency room.

I was wheeled into a room with a desk, and a lady in scrubs began asking for information. My face was swollen, and my eyes were black. My lips were bruised and swollen, my left arm was fractured, and my right leg badly bruised.

After she gathered all my insurance information, she began to ask about my injuries. When I told her that I ran into a parked car, she asked if the police had been notified and if I had been wearing a seat belt.

I explained that I had literally run into the car, and I was not driving. She questioned me several times about my injuries, then she questioned my husband, and then she questioned me again. My story was so unbelievable, she thought Jon had beaten me. Even as they began the X-rays and other treatments, she continued to try to find loopholes in my story. Jon's mom worked at the hospital, and his dad was a well-known professor. The lady with all the questions knew them both. If we had been strangers, we would have been turned over to the authorities for sure.

Finally they sent me home with some painkillers and instructions to call my family doctor in the morning. The pills did not give me much relief. I could not sleep because of the pain, so I got out of bed and sat down in the rocking chair in front of the picture window. When at last morning shed its light, I looked again toward the street where my pain had begun. I saw a dark car parked right behind a red one. The red car I had seen, but that dark car was invisible in the black of the moonless sky.

Suddenly, I caught sight of something that really scared me; there on the front fender was a huge dent. I fretted and worried about how to pay for the damages and who to call to report what I had done. When I could bear it no longer, I limped out to the curb to examine the extent of the damage. I was swept with relief when I noticed the rust and realized that I couldn't have caused the dent.

It took a number of weeks to recover fully from my injuries, but it gave me an opportunity to laugh every time I had to explain my messed-up body to someone. I found out the cast on my left arm was a perfect resting place for hot pizza pans, and I became an even more efficient waitress. Eventually the swelling went down, and the cast came off, but the jokes at my expense continued for many months, even years.

I ran into a parked car and lived to tell about it. And I'm still laughing.

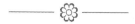

Connie and her husband, Jon, still laugh about that crazy accident and many other things that have happened in their years together. They have three children ages fourteen, sixteen, and twenty, who say it is hard to know what they really remember from their family's history and what they know because of their mom's stories.

Baking Up a Storm

Darlene A. Buechel

My parents have been through a lot in their forty-six years of marriage, including my mom's diabetes diagnosis and the scary blood clots my dad developed after his knee and hip replacement surgeries. While neither of them had a fairy-tale childhood, they vowed to provide a happy family life for my brother, sister, and me.

My dad, Eugene, did not have an easy start in life. When he was just a baby, his mother contracted tuberculosis and was sent to a sanatorium, where she later died. A few grainy black-and-white photographs are the only memories he has of Mary, his mother. Eugene does not have many memories of his father either, since he was only five when his dad, a painter, died of lead poisoning. After that, Eugene and his older brother, Melvin, were sent to an orphanage, where they spent one lonely Christmas.

Even then, Eugene had a positive attitude about his circumstances. Although each child got one orange and one toy for Christmas, he was happy to play with thirty toys, since they shared with one another. Eventually an aunt and uncle took the boys in, but they had a rough childhood and were treated more like hired hands than sons on their uncle's farm. My dad always dreamed of a family that shared and cared about each other, and he got his wish when he was blessed with his wife and three children.

My mom, Janet, also grew up on a farm and learned hard work at a young age. She worked in the fields, milking cows and taking care of her younger brother and sisters. Her parents fought all the time and eventually divorced when Janet was an adult. Her greatest wish was to be part of a family living in peace. When my parents married in 1955 they didn't have much material wealth, but they knew they wanted to build a family stronger than the one in which they had grown up.

Even though my mom did not have a peaceful childhood, she does have fond memories of learning to cook and helping her mother prepare heaping platters of food for the farm's threshing crew. She used to say that there's nothing like cooking for a bunch of hungry field hands who will eat three helpings of everything but still save room for dessert! My grandma had passed her culinary talents on to my mom, as well as her recipes for German cherry dumpling soup and the world's best custard pie. When I was growing up, our made-from-scratch suppers usually ended with a delicious dessert or two or three. I never remember Mom making only one pan of brownies or one pumpkin pie; she always made several treats at a time.

"May as well bake up a storm while the oven's hot!" she would smile as her rolling pin worked magic on another perfect crust.

My parents' uplifting attitude toward life showed up in all their actions, especially at the dinner table. Recently, a humid day turned into a tornado-watch evening. I left work at 5:00 P.M. and stopped by my parents' trailer home to return a pie pan that had boasted a yummy banana cream pie, which Mom had made for my daughter's birthday.

"Sit down a minute," Mom smiled. "I made a lemon meringue pie today."

Since lemon meringue is my all-time favorite dessert, it didn't take much arm-twisting. She cut me a huge slab but decided she would "be good" and not have any, since she has to regulate her diabetes.

I devoured my tangy treat as Mom gave me an update on my brother, who is recovering from a concussion and back injury. Dad was on a run to a local doctors' office, since he volunteers, driving patients to medical appointments. It amazes me that he'll still set foot in doctor's waiting rooms after having both knees and hips replaced since retirement. We call him the "bionic dad"!

Just before 6:00, I noticed the wind had picked up and my inherited arthritic knee was screaming, "A storm is brewing!" It was only a four-mile trip home, but I didn't want to get caught in a downpour, so I thanked Mom for the pie and sped off. It wasn't until I got home and turned on the television that I became concerned about my parents and their trailer home. I discovered that our area was in the middle of a tornado watch; everyone knows how vulnerable a trailer home is when a tornado blasts through the region.

The sky turned midnight blue, and pelting rain became marble-sized hail as tornado warnings were issued. A tornado was sighted over an area lake, making the warning more than a precaution. I felt safe in our old farmhouse, but I thanked God that my parents had their neighbor's basement to retreat to for the duration of the storm.

When the warnings and watches were cancelled at 7:30, I wanted to unwind with a good book and a tall glass of lemonade, but first I had a phone call to make. A call to Mom is never quick, since she's quite a talker, but I had to put my mind at ease and get her version of the wicked weather.

"Well, your dad got home just when the heavy rain started," Mom explained. "I'd made a good supper of barbecued chicken, twice-baked potatoes, buttered carrots, salad, and buttered broccoli, so we sat down to eat. We'd just dug in when the fire trucks came by warning people to take cover.

" 'Well, Gene, what should we do?' " I asked your dad. "And do you know what he said? 'Let's finish supper and eat our pie for dessert. If it's our time to go, at least we had a good meal and we went together!'

"So, that's what we did. We finished our supper; we enjoyed every bit of it. And see that? The storm went away, so it's a good thing we didn't waste a good meal!"

I'm sure the National Weather Service would not have approved of my parents' decision. While their neighbors were scurrying for cover in an underground cellar or basement, my mom and dad were calmly eating lemon meringue pie and listening to their cassette of polka music. Instead of worrying about whether their mobile home would get blown to Kansas, they were content to be together, enjoying their dessert and hoping for the best.

Foolish, or content? Stubborn, or at peace? Probably a little of all those things. But chances are I'll never look at lemon meringue pie quite the same again. My mom and dad have enough serenity and love to weather just about anything. Until the day they die, I hope the pies will keep on coming, served up with a heaping dose of their joy as well.

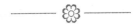

Darlene Buechel, a Wisconsin "cheese head," would like to thank her parents, Gene and Janet Totzke (from Hilbert, Wisconsin), for being fine providers of love, attention, and pie. This story is for them as they weather life's storms and toast the good times together.

No Longer the Ugly Stepmother

Deb Haggerty

Jimmy's coming to live with us! I was so excited! My husband Roy's six-year-old son was coming to live with us full-time. His mom was doing a very noble thing. Jimmy had some unique learning requirements and needed special attention and therapy—something I could help with, since I had a very flexible work schedule. Not able to have my own children, I was delighted to be able to help raise this delightful, blond-headed, happy little boy.

Over the years, little Jimmy became James. By the time he was sixteen, he was a surly, obnoxious, foul-mouthed teenager. Oh, how I wished for that cuddly boy in Doctor Dentons to return. Why did I ever think I could cope with a boy? When did he transmute into the "enemy" and I into the "ugly stepmother"?

Roy was often out of the country on business. I was coping the best I could with James, but I was really struggling.

I functioned as Mom's Taxi Service. One time James called me to pick up him and his best friend, Colin, at their favorite skateboarding place, but when I got there, no James, no Colin. Finally my cell phone rang. "Where are you, Mom?" "I'm right where you said you'd be—where are *you*?" "Oh, Colin and me decided to get a hamburger—we're down the hill at Burger King."

This scene was followed by James yelling and swearing at me when I confronted him with my frustration. The argument that followed I imagine takes place in many a stepparent's household: "As long as you are in our house, you will obey our rules!" "This is my dad's house, and I don't have to listen to you!" "I am your father's wife and I am in charge while he is gone!" "I'm leaving this f—-ing place!"

After uttering those words, James stormed downstairs to his room. In a panic, I locked the door to the downstairs and frantically called his father. What would I do if James ran away while Roy was gone?

Thank goodness I reached Roy. As calmly as I could, I explained what had happened. He asked to speak with James. I called James to the phone and left the room. Later Roy called me back and said it was okay and that he'd be home the next day. I found out when he arrived that he'd placated James and sided with him on the argument. From that point on, I had no control over James or any say in what he was or wasn't allowed to do. I felt like an unwelcome stranger in my own home.

The tension in our home continued for several years. I was a very angry and depressed person. I felt utterly and totally out of control. I knew that if it came to a choice between his son and me, my husband would choose his son.

The year James was a senior in high school, he was assigned to whom the students referred to as the "worst" English teacher. All the kids had to do a research paper, which would extend over most of the school year. Roy pleaded with me to help James with the project. "You're so good at writing—you'll know just how to help him put it together. You know how he struggles with things like this."

Flattered at being asked to help for a change, I agreed. The first part of the project was to pick a book. James picked *Deliverance*. Then he picked a thesis and scoured the library and the Internet for research. The night before his research cards were due, he was up until 3:00 A.M. finishing them. He then drove them to a friend's house for her to deliver in class, since we were going away on a trip and he had an excused absence. When he returned to class after the trip, the teacher ridiculed him about having someone else turn in his cards: "You just wanted to play hooky!"

The outline and thesis statement were next. James and I worked for hours to get it just right. Finally, I went to bed while he finished up. The next morning, I found on my desk one of the rewards a stepmother often dreams of but seldom receives. A letter from James read, "Mom, thanks so much for helping me on this project. I just know that we'll get a really high grade on it. There isn't any way to tell you how much I appreciate it. Love, your son, James."

I cried as I showed Roy the letter.

We anxiously awaited his grade on the outline—it came back "0"! And next to his thesis statement was the scrawl, "Who cares?" James was demoralized, and I was furious! "What kind of a teacher is this? Does he call this a critique? How is James supposed to know what he's done wrong? And besides, there isn't anything wrong with this!"

My husband was equally incensed. He wanted to head into school to confront the teacher. James told us about all the negative and slanderous comments the teacher had been making about him in front of the class as well as several inappropriate stories the teacher had told the students. "In fact," James told us, "several times he's said in front of the class that no matter what I do, I'm not going to pass!"

Now deadly calm, I told my husband that confronting this particular teacher would not help—I would go and talk to the principal.

A day later I was in the principal's office armed with my arguments on James's behalf. The principal made the major mistake of trying to patronize me. I assured him that I knew what I was talking about—that I'd been an English major in college and had an M.B.A., in addition to being a published author. He backpedaled frantically. I told him we wanted James transferred to another section of English with a different teacher. He assured me that was not possible and that James had probably just overreacted. This teacher, he related, was one of the best, though on the tough side.

I queried him if he thought constructive criticism was part of a teacher's job on a project such as this. "Oh, it's one of the most important parts!" "Then explain to me how this fits with constructive criticism?" I showed him the outline with the teacher's comment. "And let me show you how James felt about it before he got this back." I showed him my prized letter.

Crestfallen, the principal allowed there was nothing constructive in the comments James had been given. I repeated our desire to have James transferred. He reiterated that it was not possible. I told him that all James needed to graduate was a passing grade in English. I was not going to allow him to prevent my son from graduating, even if I had to pull James out of school and home-school him! I further informed the principal that I was sure the P.T.A. would love to hear about this teacher and that I would find other parents who were willing to testify to the treatment their kids had received when in this teacher's class. Finally he capitulated: "All right, Mrs. Haggerty. We'll move James to another class."

While relating my conversation to Roy and James later, I could see the incredulity on James's face. His stepmom had done the impossible! No one went up against this teacher and won—no one had ever been transferred out, despite frequent attempts. At that point a transformation occurred in our relationship. I started to see James as a person trying very hard to succeed, given the obstacles he had to overcome. He started to see me as a person who loved him and really wanted to help and to be a part of his life.

While James's and my relationship did not become smooth overnight, things did improve. Today he's a bright young man earnestly working to be a success at his job. I received my latest "reward" just recently. James is building his first house. "Mom, will you come and meet with the designer with me to pick out the options? You're so good at that." We spent a delightful morning doing the planning for his house and then had a very gracious lunch.

I now see my son as a very special person and not the "enemy." He now sees me as a friend and not the "wicked stepmother." In fact, the birthday card I got from him this year reads: "For My Mother. One kindness follows another, and you are the source. You give advice when it's asked for, encouragement when it's needed, and kindness when it means the most. I hope you'll always know how much that means to me." Yes, James, I know. I hope you know how much you mean to me. I am proud to be considered your mother. You have been one of the greatest challenges of my life, and you have also been one of its greatest rewards.

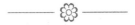

Deb Haggerty is an author and speaker who lives in Orlando, Florida, with her husband, Roy, and Cocoa the dog. Deb is a three-year breast cancer survivor and is actively working through her speaking and the Florida Breast Cancer Coalition to educate women and help eradicate the disease. James is now living and working in Jacksonville, Florida, for Ajilon Consulting and enjoys racecar driving and golf.

Never Poor in Spirit

Donna Martin McMahon

*P*overty does not have to be a miserable experience. My family has taught me that most of the blessings in life have nothing to do with money.

On June 24, 1900, more than one hundred years ago, a baby girl was born to a young couple in the backwoods country of Seminole, Oklahoma. Cordie and John Brown were very proud of their firstborn and invited the neighbors to come and welcome little Lavonia Bell to the world. One of Cordie's closest neighbors and her good friend, Nancy Jane Martin, had a boy named Oren, the last of thirteen children, who was only three years old at the time. When he saw the new baby lying on her mother's lap, he lifted himself up ever so carefully and gave her a kiss on the forehead.

Lavonia's father, John Brown, was a farmer and raised and trained hunting dogs to supplement the income from his farm. Oren's father, Leonadis Martin, was a blacksmith by trade, and he was ambidextrous. This enabled him to pick up a hammer with either hand and use it equally well. He was very good at his trade, but life was hard and work was scarce. A few years went by, and the families moved apart out of necessity.

Even living apart, the families still kept in contact and would help each other whenever possible. In about 1910, Cordie and John Brown decided to move to the Kiamichi Mountains in southeastern Oklahoma, where their friends now lived. John knew that the trip would be long and difficult and that help would be needed for herding the cattle along the way, so he enlisted the aid of some of the older boys in the Martin family.

There was a covered wagon for their food and personal belongings and another wagon to carry the feed for the animals. Each night the families would stop and make camp and each day press on toward the mountains.

Lavonia Bell, now about ten years old, would walk for a while and then, when she was tired, would ride in a wagon. It took her and her family about two weeks on the trail to make the trip, but all went well and they arrived safely.

As time went on, Lavonia and Oren, now eighteen and twenty-one, having known each other all their lives, fell in love. One day as Lavonia was sitting on the woodpile swinging her feet, she saw Oren riding up the dirt road on his horse. He got off, sat on the pile of wood with her, and asked her to be his wife. She accepted, and they were married on May 11, 1919, a day that would later fall many times on what we now know as Mother's Day.

For a wedding present, he was able to buy her a rolling pin, broom, washboard, and pot to start out their housekeeping. They were happy and hardworking and loved children. Even when older, they were like flirtatious lovers. Oren would catch her in the kitchen with her hands in sudsy dishwater and would take that opportunity to untie her apron strings, while giving her a friendly pat on her backside and a hug from behind. Lavonia was always ready to help him in any way she could and was his strongest supporter in every challenge life brought their way.

I am the youngest of their ten children. We were poor, but Mom and Dad never let us know it. In the winter, after the second good snow, we made snow ice cream with fresh ingredients from our farm. Then we'd sit around a fat potbellied woodstove in the living room devouring huge bowls, while shivering as we asked for more. The word *bored* was not in our vocabulary.

In the spring we would walk behind Dad as he and our horse plowed the field, and we would drop and cover the seeds for long rows of corn, peas, and other vegetables that Mom and we would later can for our winter foods. On days when our work was done, we would follow Mother through the woods, being as quiet as possible, in hopes that we would find a new bird nest or see a couple of gray squirrels chasing each other around an old oak tree. Then we would sit on a rock, with our feet in the creek, watching crawdads back up quickly to get out of our way.

In the summer, when we could afford it, we would buy a block of ice from the ice dock and churn up a big freezer of homemade ice cream. The younger kids would take turns sitting on the top of the gunnysacks covering the salt and chunks of ice, while one of the older kids turned the crank until it could be turned no more. Then to further cool off his rowdy crew, Dad would pile everyone in the pickup and take us for a swim at the ponds made by the removal of gravel from the gravel pits, where we would swim and play late into the warm summer night. Many were the times only the darkness could make us abandon the fun and go home.

In the fall, we would pick up hickory nuts, walnuts, and pecans to crack during those long winter evenings. Always there were friends, and lots of aunts, uncles, and cousins with whom to share our lives. Most of the adults played some kind of musical instrument, from banjos, fiddles, and guitars to spoons, Jew's harps, and washboards. There were lots of songs, dancing, and fun times to help the family over the hard places in the road. For the most part, life was good.

Mom and Dad lived together for sixty-one years before he died, and she lived on for another twenty-two years without him until her death in March 2002. She was just three months shy of her one hundred and second birthday, and her life had spanned three generations. They brought ten children into the world, and had thirty-one grandchildren, sixty-nine great-grandchildren, and more than forty-one great-great-grandchildren.

Their greatest legacy was in showing us how to find the best things in life even during adversity. They taught us to love our neighbor as ourselves and to love God above all else. We learned that being poor by the world's standards did not make us poor in hope, joy, and spirit. Most of all, they taught us that the old adage, "the best things in life are free," is absolutely true. That is a gift no amount of money can buy.

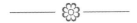

Donna McMahon lives in northern California with Frank, her husband of forty-five years. They have two daughters and sons-in-law, two grandsons, and one granddaughter. Donna is part of a vocal team, along with her daughter and grandson, at church, as well as being a classroom teacher. She has tried to instill in her children and grandchildren the joys of music and the beauty of the handiwork of the Great Master Artist.

Donna's mother was indeed very special. On her one-hundredth birthday, she was taken out to a Chinese restaurant, and during dinner she put down her fork and began singing "Amazing Grace." The cooks and waitresses came out of the kitchen, the people in the restaurant put down their forks, and everyone listened to her sweet voice. At her memorial service that song was sung, especially for her.

Lavender Walls

Freda Douglas

As a young woman growing up in the late 1940s and early '50s, I was socialized to give in to the whims of my husband.

When I married for the first time, my husband not only picked out my clothes—and I let him, because it was easier to wear what he liked—he also picked out the colors for decorating our home. When we painted the house yellow with brown trim, I really wanted it white with barn-red trim, but I had no say in the matter.

Only once in our marriage did I assert myself about color. We owned a restaurant (he picked the décor for that, too), and I kept the books and records for the restaurant at home. We had a large house with three bedrooms, so I took over the back bedroom for my office. You could have heard the explosion across the river when my husband came home from his job at the radio station and discovered I had painted the walls of my office lavender, the ceiling and woodwork white, with robin-egg blue and white café curtains, all of which went nicely with the dark blue rug and dark blue sofa bed.

He sputtered and fumed. By nature I was very pliant when it came to my husband, but I'd had enough. I stomped my foot and declared, "This is *my* office. When you decide to take over the bookwork for the pizza shop, I don't care what color you paint the office. But as long as I do the work, I pick the paint!" When we later sold the house, the office was still lavender.

Probably because Mother was very domineering with Daddy, and I saw many times how her personality had hurt him, I vowed to not be domineering with my husband. After twenty-three years of marriage, my husband, Rollie, went to be with his Maker. I was alone for about two years before I met, and fell in love with, the man who became my second husband, John.

I was fifty years young when I married John. The world had changed for women by then; all around me, women were asserting themselves more. But even though my second husband was very different from my first, I continued to be compliant with him, and once again, I catered to his likes and dislikes. Of course, we decorated our home according to his style.

After seventeen years of marriage John was diagnosed with a particularly virulent form of cancer. He was put to rest two months later. I was devastated. I was sixty-eight by that time, and not at all prepared to be a widow. My doctor diagnosed me with clinical depression and prescribed medication. The medicine did its job and helped me to function again, but I still had to deal with *me*.

I sold our car, which I didn't need because I no longer drove as the result of a stroke I had in 1994. I put the money in my money market account, so I wouldn't be inclined to spend it. The money sat there until friends of mine, Arlene and Butch, returned for the winter to the retirement village where I live. I shared with them an earth-shattering decision I had made, after nearly seven months since John had died. My history with the men in my life explains why this was such a big deal.

I decided to change the décor of the house. I needed to put my personality into it. Everywhere I turned I was seeing John. I needed to find myself again. I sat with Arlene and Butch around the dining room table, and we discussed the changes I wanted to make in my house. Butch, a handy guy and a good friend, agreed to do the work for me. I can't tell you how excited I was. It was the first joy I had felt in many months.

When Butch and his friends finished the house, pink and gray ceramic tiles replaced the rugs in the kitchen and dining area, and the divider between the kitchen and dining room was removed. The breakfast booth and table were replaced with a custom-made ceramic tabletop, which Butch installed high enough for me to be able to use my wheelchair comfortably. The white walls, which John had preferred, were repainted a pale, but very distinct, lavender (ah, wouldn't my first husband be screaming—a lavender living room!).

The biggest change was made in the master bathroom. The rug was replaced with maroon ceramic tile, with coordinating tile set on point. Setting the tiles on point, as opposed to laying them square, dramatically improved the look of the floor. The walls, which had always been wallpapered, were painted white with a sponge chair rail of lavender. A new carpet was installed. The effect was astonishing. My spirits were extraordinarily lifted: it was a redecorating of my home and a release of my spirit at the same time.

I am finally living in *my* home. Memories, especially good memories like I had with John, are wonderful to keep as long as they are kept in perspective. Since the remodeling and restoration of my home, my will not only to live, but to prosper, has also been restored. I can feel the spirit of hope, and yes, even love for life, resonate throughout every room in this home, now shared by my cat and me.

The medication helped ease my depression, but a can of paint—yes, lavender—and the permission I gave myself to design my own home, just for me, did wonders more.

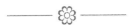

Freda Douglas still lives in the retirement village where she and John moved in 1984. She keeps busy writing her weekly newspaper column and running her Internet businesses.

I'm Still Standing!

Barbara Hammack

When I tell you my story, it will sound so gruesome that you'll wonder what it's doing in a book entitled *Half Full*. I am only fifty-six but more battered by life than I ever could have imagined. But I have reached the promised land. I am strong, confident, and optimistic, even though, looking back at the past fifteen years, I don't know why I am still standing, laughing, or even living. I am a survivor!

My so-called charmed life began to unravel when my father died from cancer in 1987. One year later, my mother was diagnosed with cancer and died fifteen months later. During that time, my marriage turned out to be not so wonderful, and my husband and I separated shortly after my mother died. Soon after that, the man I had almost married in college—my true soul mate and love of my life—reappeared. After a short, blissful reunion, he left me in 1991, shortly after I was diagnosed with cancer.

I was diagnosed with "smoldering" multiple myeloma, an incurable cancer of the plasma cells; at that time there were very few options for treatment, and the prognosis was pessimistic. I was the glue holding my adolescent kids together, since their dad was recovering from the severe depression that had destroyed our marriage. I had to live for them, period.

In 1994, when my cancer stopped "smoldering" and required aggressive treatment if I were to survive, I agreed to have a bone marrow and stem cell transplant, with the hope of buying more years. It worked. I was able to see each of my children graduate from both high school and college, and I fully intend to see my son's graduation from law school in 2003.

My journey since 1994 has not been easy. Though I recovered from the transplant and was able to return to work, I suffered a severe shingles outbreak in 1995, which left me with permanent intermittent neuropathic pain that can make moving difficult. I also had a very difficult time recovering when my college sweetheart left me. He and I reconnected briefly in 1996, but that ended with no closure, and we never talked again to resolve things.

It was only by chance that as I skimmed the obituaries one night in September 1999, I read that my former sweetheart had died a lonely death from esophageal cancer. His death devastated me, even though we were no longer together. I slipped into the deepest of depressions as I entered a forced retirement, on disability, owing to my ongoing health problems.

Those six months of intense grief work were the most important months of my life. I searched, and found, my spiritual center. I listened to people who described near-death experiences and was comforted and inspired by their spiritual experiences. I joined a group of cancer survivors in meditation and guided imagery sessions. I continued working with my beloved therapist, who has been with me through all my battles. I swam. I walked and connected with nature. I sought to find meaning in all the losses that I had experienced.

Slowly, I began to feel renewed. The days when I focused on me, and my pain and sadness, were empty, but the days when I connected with other people left me feeling alive and joyful.

Now, with so much behind me, I walk with an air of confidence. Though I was diagnosed with two additional illnesses in November of 2001—type II diabetes and ocular myasthenia gravis (a degenerative muscular condition), I am fortunate that both of these conditions are under control. I've lost many of the extra pounds I'd put on, and have reinvented my life to adapt to my health needs and limitations. I choose to focus on what I *can* do. This has made all the difference.

I attend a meditation group. I tutor two girls from other countries as they adjust to a new culture. I consult for the agency that used to employ me. I counsel newly diagnosed myeloma patients, both by phone and through an on-line support group. I write a quarterly column called "A Survivor's Perspective" for the Life with Cancer Center, a nonprofit group. I lunch a few days a week with old and new friends. I play bridge. I attend educational programs for people over fifty-five. And, of course, there are my children.

When people tell me that I am an inspiration to them, and that they could never have handled what I have, I repeat the wise advice given to me so many years ago by my memorable student, Barbara, a sixty-year-old woman who reassured me, when I confessed that I didn't know how I would cope with the losses that often come with aging, by saying: "One of the joys of being sixty years old is that I have been tested by life. Now that I have passed some of these tests, I am no longer afraid."

I, too, am no longer afraid. I laugh every day and cry only when necessary. Life is good.

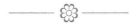

Barbara Hammack currently lives in Kensington, Maryland, with her daughter, her son's cat, and much of his unused furniture while he finishes law school at Columbia University. She volunteers with immigrant children and other at-risk students and with multiple myeloma cancer patients. Her favorite place to be is at the beach. She is a lifelong educator, with a master's in human development. At times she feels like her hobby is going to doctors, but she feels blessed to have a wonderful medical team available as needed.

Interrupted Love

Jaime Strauss Sefton

*I*was still young when my husband died from a heart attack—uninsured, leaving me lonely and devastated with two sons to raise. I had always worked, but now I would have to devote more time to my counseling practice and officiate at more weddings, christenings, and funerals as a minister in Australia, where I live.

I didn't officiate at my husband's funeral, but I should have. The appointed minister stepped too near to the edge of the grave and almost fell in. He forgot my husband's name and couldn't find his glasses to read his notes. My sons were ready to put the minister in his own grave, but the farce lightened the atmosphere, and I knew my spouse would have laughed, too.

The years passed: lonely, hard-working years. The boys left home and found employment in distant cities. They went where the work was, and they prospered. I was very proud. I dated, but unsuccessfully. Little by little, after many years, I gave up on remarrying.

The Internet was a godsend. I chatted and wrote to others online, and my isolated world began to open up. And then I got the email that was to change my life. I was "found" by the first boy I had ever dated and loved, who was living in England. We excitedly exchanged phone numbers by email, and he called me immediately, at 4:30 in the morning.

Almost incoherent from the excitement of finding me, he explained that he had nursed his wife through cancer, and that prior to her passing, she had insisted that he make a new life for himself. He had recently learned from meeting old friends of mine that I was widowed and living in Australia, and he asked if he could come to Australia to meet me.

"I had a happy marriage," he said, "but you were always in my heart. I was a boy when I asked to marry you, and you chose a sophisticated man over me. I couldn't blame you. But if you're willing to see me, I'll book the first available flight."

Waiting at the airport, a few days later, I decided I must be mad. I had no idea what he would look like now. We were teens when our romance flourished. I hadn't changed too much in appearance, but some people do. How on earth would I recognize him?

The busy concourse looked like Times Square on New Year's Eve. There were men of every shape and description. I scanned only those with pale, English skins. None of them looked right. And then, suddenly, a tall, tanned, dark-haired man was standing in front of me, laughing.

I had agonized about how I was to greet him, but our hug was spontaneous and felt just right. After our long separation, incredibly, we just took up where we had left off. Ten days later, in a cable car over the Cairns hinterland, with the sparkling turquoise sea in the background, Laurence asked me to marry him.

I said, "Yes!" without hesitation. Our idyllic holiday ended all too soon when he flew back to England to settle his affairs and provide Australian immigration with the necessary information. Because he was associated with an Australian company in England, moving to Australia would give him the new life he wanted and new business opportunities.

I amazed family and friends with my transforming news and immediately started planning our wedding, which was scheduled for Laurence's return in sixteen weeks, to satisfy the legalities. As I was determined to officiate my own marriage, we would have a brief ceremony at the courthouse, and a few weeks later, a service and formal reception with invited guests.

A short while before Laurence's return, scheduled for two days before we married, I underwent some oral surgery that could not wait. To my horror, it resulted in accidental bruising to my whole face. The slightest touch made me wince. I even had to sleep sitting up!

"You won't even be able to kiss me; what kind of honeymoon is that?" I mumbled painfully during our telephone conversations.

"So, I'll kiss the other bits of you," Laurence reassured me.

We decided not to postpone the wedding. We had waited thirty years for one another. We weren't going to wait another week. Once again, I was at the airport. I was very self-conscious about my stiff face, but one look at Laurence's made me forget all about it. He looked positively green and was sweating with fever. I stopped at the first pharmacy I saw, plied him with pills, and packed him off to bed as soon as we reached home. There he stayed until the morning we had to go to the court.

He barely held it together during our celebratory lunch, then he was back in bed until two days later, when we set off for our week-long honeymoon on a tropical island. It was a total disaster! Not only was he ill the entire time, but it was the hottest summer for a hundred years and, coming from freezing England, the heat and humidity wiped out whatever slight energy he could muster to get out of bed.

Back home, we went ahead with preparations for our second wedding, to which family and friends were coming from overseas.

"We'll have a proper second honeymoon," Laurence promised.

"It doesn't matter," I said. "Just having you here, and being married and loved, is all I need."

As with all weddings, there was the usual last-minute flurry and panic, but I felt confident all would be right on the day.

With one week to go, my face had finally healed, Laurence was fighting fit, and we were determined to get our marriage off to the right start. And that was when we discovered ... the lump. Not pea sized or like a grain of rice, *no*, it was a 3/4-inch protuberance in my breast that had come completely out of nowhere! Like all health-conscious women, I had been self-examining each month and had felt nothing.

Laurence was stoic, but I was furious. He had lost his first wife to cancer; he didn't need this. He'd just found me; he didn't want to lose me again, and I wanted to hold on to the happiness I had rediscovered. Breast cancer was *not* on the guest list.

The medical system worked fast and efficiently. My doctor referred me, at once, to the hospital and I underwent mammography, ultrasound, and biopsy and was face-to-face with the oncology surgeon two days later. "You're critical," he said quietly.

"We're having our wedding this weekend, and I have overseas visitors to show around," I answered, my practical and organizational mind whirling.

"I'll let you have the wedding and a couple of days, then I operate," he said firmly.

I looked at my frozen husband. "We are going to tell no one and make this the best, fun-filled wedding ever," I vowed, and we did. Everyone, my sons especially, were thrilled that my loneliness was over. I had reunited with my childhood sweetheart—what a fairy tale! We gave it everything we had, postponing any thoughts about the future.

A few days later, I gave Laurence a big hug and went to be prepped for surgery. I felt the timing was extraordinary. Did God send me Laurence when he did so I wouldn't have to go through this on my own? I couldn't help but wonder.

The surgeon found the lump encapsulated, so I was able to keep the majority of my breast. Lymph nodes, which they removed from under my arm, were cancer free, but as a precautionary measure, I went through weeks of radiation. I was sore and sorry, and my new husband had to keep his distance, but at least we were together. We bought a house and moved in the day before reporting to the hospital for treatment. As I lay beneath the X-ray equipment, I thought about my recent marriage to Laurence and allowed myself to imagine our new life together and refused to obsess about death. I couldn't believe that God would reunite us after all these years only to separate us so swiftly.

I was supposed to take things easy, but there was so much to do. Our boxes were still unpacked, when suddenly Laurence's daughter announced she was getting married, in London, a few days after my radiotherapy was to finish. Forty-eight hours after I eased myself off the treatment table, we boarded the plane. As I had been forewarned, the cumulative blistering and peeling on my chest intensified, and sleeping was a problem, but I was alive.

We left icy England for a stopover in Malaysia involving a taxi that broke down and a driver who left us to broil in the fierce sun for an hour. We arrived back in Australia with raging temperatures. It was more than two weeks before we took our heads out of the tissue boxes and felt strong enough to venture outside for more than a few minutes. Sharing the flu together was not how we had hoped to get a fresh start on our marriage.

A few days after we began to feel better, the weather was perfect. "Let's explore our land," I said excitedly. "We only know the boundaries of our fifty-six acres, not the area in detail."

Using the four-wheel-drive, clearing the scrub bush as we went, was great fun. On my fourth descent from the pickup, as I went to remove a dead branch, my right leg plunged deeply into a concealed burrow. The sudden nothingness and jarring flung me face down on the ground. Waves of pain swept through my twisted foot and knee. Although nothing was broken, Laurence had to lift me back up into the vehicle and drive me home. The swelling and stiffness in my leg intensified, and it was a long while before I could walk without a stick or get my foot back into a shoe.

As a minister, officiating weddings, how many times had I used the words "in sickness and in health"?

Laurence and I are hoping that we've gotten all the sickness part of our life out of the way, early on. The adversity we have shared since our reunion has given us the kind of strength and togetherness that often takes a marriage many years to achieve. We have learned to laugh together, because, sometimes, when things are so bad, all you can do is laugh—it *is* the best medicine. Our love has withstood the test of time, and we are now looking forward to our future together.

Last week, at his immigration medical, Laurence was told by the physician that he has tuberculosis. We laughed. What else is there to do?

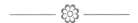

Jaime and Laurence are living each day as it comes. They are enjoying their Australian bush home, which they share with one cat, two horses, five chooks (chickens), and several kangaroos and wallabies. They are landscaping the scrub land into beautiful gardens, where Jaime has begun to hold weddings. She counsels in a sunroom overlooking the gardens, and she knows it helps her clients feel better. Both Jaime and Laurence are having regular checkups. Thank God, so far both are okay. They're too busy to be ill—and they love each other! That's what matters.

Getting Fired Got Me Fired Up

Jeff Gross

*A*t one time in my life, I might have thought that getting fired from a job would be too devastating for my ego to handle. But as things go, the fiasco of my earlier failed years turned out to be the greatest impetus for my success later in life. Who knows; if I hadn't gotten fired, maybe I'd still be working in a job I hated, dreaming about what could have been.

I can vividly recall the tasteless monologue I delivered more than twenty years ago, which eventually got me canned from my first real job. I was an immature and sarcastic young college graduate working in the "toiletry department" as a department manager. To the horror and disbelief of the other department managers who witnessed my Machiavellian display of employment hara-kiri, it went something like this: "This week's best-seller comes from the toiletry department. It is Fluffy toilet paper. As a matter of fact, we are thinking of changing the name of the drug department to the fantasy department, because where else in the whole store can you tell the customer to take the merchandise and stick it!" The room was filled with a deadly silence. It was as if I was taunting my boss, à la Clint Eastwood in his famous showdown: "Go ahead, make my day."

Surprisingly, that tirade did not lead to my immediate termination. It was suggested, though, at my next performance review, that my talents might be better suited elsewhere. Furthermore, I had ninety days to clean up my act, or I would be asked to leave. I was devastated by the prospect of leaving on their terms, not mine. None of my career plans included failure. It certainly was not part of the romantic vision of "work hard and climb the corporate ladder" ideology to which I had naively subscribed when I left college.

Luckily, I found another job relatively quickly, so I did get to leave my position on my own terms. I returned from Saint Louis to my hometown of Minneapolis, reinvigorated and more determined than ever to make my mark on the business world. This new "marriage" also ended in divorce after four years. Again, I was left to pick up the pieces—of my career and self-esteem. At least that was the only new marriage that ended in divorce, though I am sure my bride of one week had plenty of second thoughts when my job ended.

After some lengthy introspection, I came to the conclusion that the only real job security I could count on was working for myself. This ultimately led to a ten-year foray in the fast-food business. I complemented my bachelor's degree with a self-proclaimed "master's in mayo" to learn how to make sandwiches and four weeks of "sundae school" to learn the finer points of the ice cream business. When my growth plateaued, a mid-life "evaluation" triggered my exit from the culinary service world. A 1,400-mile trek with my family to the East Coast would begin a new adventure. This time, I would be a franchisee for a national chain of hair salons.

Reflecting back on the two decades since I graduated from the University of Wisconsin, I have a better appreciation of the divergent paths careers can take. Perhaps colleges will someday offer a course in "Surviving Screwups" in conjunction with classes on résumé writing and interviewing. I could have benefited from such a class. But now, I could teach it. And in truth, my life is better because of these experiences. Even my beloved and patient wife would now agree.

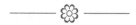

Jeff Gross lives with his wife, Marci, sons Noah and Zachary, and their five-pound guard dog, Schmutzik. They are adjusting to and enjoying life on the East Coast and continue to grow personally and professionally.

Walking Trellis

Jennifer Oliver

*I*n seventh grade, a group of us positioned our desks in a circle to work on a team assignment. Like all kids that age, we joked more than we worked on the task at hand. At one point I made a facetious comment to a very cute boy, "Yeah, yeah, Paul. And you're a dog."

He was unfamiliar with my sense of humor, and his backlash startled me.

"Oh, yeah? Well, *you're* the dog!"

Silence. Complete, utter silence. I slunk down in my chair, my face on fire from the pity directed at me, tears burning in my eyes.

Well, of course. I was a dog in the sense that I suffered from acute acne, wore bug-eyed glasses and hearing aids, and had thin hair that would not yield to a curling iron. But still. It hurt that no one came to my defense.

My dogness was reinforced by a party I went to not long after that incident. The excitement over attending my very first boy-girl party was overshadowed as soon as I arrived on Roseanne's doorstep with my best friend.

"Hey, Dee Dee!" Roseanne greeted my friend. "I have the perfect guy for you!"

I stood by while Roseanne greeted each girl with the name of her dancing partner. Everyone, that is, except me. While one slow song after another filled the darkened living room, I perched expectantly on the couch with a plastic smile. Sipping soda, I watched each couple make out while swaying to the tunes. I hoped against hope someone would come up for air long enough to ask me to dance.

No one did.

During one Girl Scouts meeting, a woman from a cosmetics company paid a visit to our troupe. I colored my face with a wealth of eye shadow, foundation, mascara, rouge ... the whole nine yards. When I turned to face my giggling girlfriends, their response was music to my ears, even if I was hard of hearing.

"Jennifer! You look bee-yoo-ti-ful!"

No one had ever said that to me before. I floated home that night.

"Dad," I said, snuggling up to him in front of the late-night news. "When can I start wearing makeup?"

"Never," was his wry response. "You're beautiful just the way you are. Besides, you're only thirteen." Dads were obviously clueless.

I stared for hours at Olivia Newton-John's album covers. Both she and Farrah Fawcett were, in my mind, icons of beauty with porcelain complexions and luxurious hair. I prayed and prayed I would be the one ugly duckling that turned into swans like them.

When I was a freshman in high school, my mother lengthened the leash. I splurged and spent all my allowance on makeup. Frosted blue eye shadow, strawberry lip gloss, plum blush, brown-black mascara, ivory foundation. I learned how to curl my hair so that it feathered back just like Farrah's. I began to wear contacts. With all this makeup, my acne was not as noticeable. For the first time in my life, I faced the world with confidence.

With both confidence and humor on my side, I bloomed into a swan. Yet not once did I lose sight of my roots as an ugly duckling. I was friendly to everyone, mingling with the popular kids, and the ones who were more isolated. Boys started to take notice. My dancing card filled quickly.

Then one day, in my senior year of high school, I stood in front of a pep assembly with a slew of girls. We were all competing for the title of Miss Prom Queen. Me! In a beauty contest! I smiled broadly as I posed in a modest dress of earth tones.

I was suddenly self-conscious of all the eyes on me, judging me. I cast my eyes down, afraid to see their smirks and finger-pointing. Surely they could see right through my makeup and know me for who I really was.

A dog.

When it came time to vote, I couldn't bear to mark the little box next to my own name. I ended up not winning the coveted title, losing by only two votes. But I was ecstatic. This was a victory!

Yet an even sweeter victory lay in store for me. I was chosen as Choir Sweetheart for the big prom night. My mother sewed my gown, its shimmering green bringing out the light in my hazel-blue eyes while I strolled down the red carpet along with the Prom Queen's entourage. As my boyfriend and I swayed under a mirrored globe to a slow song by Earth, Wind & Fire, I felt like a princess in a fairy tale.

When I was in college, I began dating Stephen, and we fell in love. One night shortly after I moved into his place, I was taking a shower. Stephen stepped into the shower.

"Stephen!" I shrieked, flicking water at him. "Get out of here!"

"What? I just want to have some fun!"

"But you can't see me like this!"

"Like what?"

I began sobbing.

"What's the matter with you?" he quizzed me.

"I don't have any makeup on," I said, my voice muffled by the hands over my face.

"Jennifer, you can be such an idiot sometimes," he said, laughing. He hugged me hard. We stood there in the shower, soapy rivulets running down our bodies.

Stephen plied my hands away.

"Let me see your face."

I lifted my face to him with my eyes squeezed shut. What he did next made me tremble.

He kissed my face, lightly, over and over again. And then, I really got it.

Stephen loved me for who I was. Like my Dad, he thought I was beautiful, without all the makeup.

Nearly five years later my roommate became my soul mate in an impromptu ceremony before a justice of the peace. Here we are, going on sixteen years now. Even after four children, Stephen still kisses my face.

Not long ago, I met my family of five after work at a Chinese restaurant. I wore my favorite dress with huge roses splashed all over it. I looked like a walking trellis.

"Mom! You look beautiful!" Cody, one of our gorgeous children, gushed.

"Yeah! You look like a giant flower!" quipped his brother, Matthew.

I'm catching the eye of younger men. And that's quite all right by me.

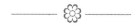

Hailing from Killeen, Texas, Jennifer Oliver is wife to awesome househubby, Stephen, and mother to four beautiful blessings, and she works full-time for the government on the side. She delivers uplifting stories through her weekly e-zine *Stories of Heart* and has been published in the *Heartwarmers* series, *Chicken Soup*, and *Stories for a Woman's Heart* series. She cites her family as her wellspring of inspiration.

Another Miracle, Not My Own

Jennifer Basye Sander

*I*t was a beautiful, clear spring day when my best friend of ten years, Laura, called to say that she was dying. "The doctors say it is in my brain now, and it won't take much longer."

She was thirty-seven years old, the mother of two young children. For once, the doctors were right. She died the following November. It didn't take long.

"It wasn't supposed to turn out this way!" I shouted at God. Laura should have had a miracle. Damn it, she deserved a miracle.

She was first diagnosed with breast cancer at age thirty-two, a shockingly young age for such a vicious disease. The younger you are, the more virulent the cancer can be. When Laura first told me her news, I, being a published writer, sat down to write an inspirational novel for her. In my novel, she was a character who'd had cancer many years before, a strong and resilient woman who'd beaten the odds and survived.

Although I may still finish that novel, even though Laura didn't make it, I soon put it aside and embarked on a slightly more practical plan. Along with Jamie Miller, another friend of Laura's, I began to work on collecting stories about Christmas miracles. Not only would a collection of Christmas miracle tales find an audience, I thought, but it will also bring in some money, something Laura and her husband could use for peace of mind.

Jamie and I interviewed many people who had experienced miracles at Christmastime, and then we wrote up their stories. Laura kept track of the administrative end of the project, and we produced a book for William Morrow, *Christmas Miracles: Magical True Stories of Modern-Day Miracles*, that became a national best-seller.

How wonderful it was to be able to spread the word about the incredible things that can happen when we open our hearts and believe. Interview after interview convinced me that miracles are everywhere, if we just open our eyes to the mystery of life.

I had a secret goal during the miracle book project. I believed with all my heart that if Laura were involved in this miracle project, if she lived and breathed the idea of miracles day in and day out, if she helped to spread the word that miracles can and do happen, then she too would be given a miracle. The hand of God was everywhere in these tales. We believed that same hand would reach down to allow her to stay with her children, to be the mother they needed her to be. Laura should earn the miracle she deserved because of our good work with the book.

Our one book turned into a series of five books on miracles. But all the while, as our books grew more popular and we gathered more tales of miracles, Laura grew sicker. Five years after she was first diagnosed, she died.

In the months following Laura's death I was furious with God. Why, after all of the good that Laura had done in her life, did God allow her to die? Why didn't she get her miracle?

The answer came to me on another clear spring day, an eerie twin to the day that Laura had called with her devastating news the year before. As I looked out my office window at the blooming azaleas, the astralillies hanging heavy from the weight of their flowers, I suddenly realized that there had been a miracle for Laura after all. I hadn't noticed the miracle of the last few years, because it wasn't the one I wanted.

I wanted Laura to live. That was what I was asking from God, and anything less was unacceptable. But God knew all along that Laura would die, so God gave her the miracle she would need. She would need help with her children, so he gave her a circle of friends to pitch in. She and her husband would need help with their finances, so he sent the miracle books project and allowed her to earn an income that would not require her to spend time away from her children in her final years of life. She would not live long, so he gave her a way to have an impact far greater than most people have in their first three decades. Her name will live on in her books, and even after her death she will continue to inspire others in their time of need.

God gave her the miracle Laura needed, even if it wasn't the one I had asked for. I am grateful that I finally saw it.

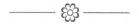

Jennifer Basye Sander lives in Granite Bay, California, with her husband and two young sons. The co-author of the *Miracles* series, she continues to look for the miracles in everyday life.

Emmy and Sara

Karin Kasdin

When Emily died, three townships mourned. She died unexpectedly from asthma at the age of nineteen, and her dream of being a dancer on Broadway has been eternally mingled with all the unfulfilled dreams of all the children taken from us for reasons we can't begin to understand.

Emily was a ballerina, with a Lilliputian body, fragile lungs, and gargantuan strength. Watching her dance was like watching the birth of a baby or the aurora borealis. Ironically, her magic took your breath away. People who watched her award-winning performances could only speak in tongues afterward.

At the time of her death, as a student at the University of Pennsylvania, Emily was contemplating a career in medicine so she could bring relief to children suffering from asthma. She would have assuaged people's pain with equal helpings of music and medicine. Her funeral, held at a synagogue that easily seats eight hundred, was standing room only.

Other daughters will be loved as much as Emily was. No daughter will ever be loved more. Other parents will grieve as exhaustively as Emily's parents did. But it would be impossible for any parents' grief to be greater. At Emily's burial her mother emitted a cry that scared the birds into silence and every other mother into immobility. Unable to run, we thought only of running. Running home to grasp our living children, to feel their breath and imbibe their energy.

The pain in that small square of graveside green seemed weighty enough to pull us all down into the ground with Emmy. Any parent present who had not already been permanently changed by the death of some other child was altered forever by this passing.

Within months after Emily's death and well into their forties, these bereft people who were already parenting an equally bereft young son, Andy, adopted a four-month-old baby girl.

I'd be surprised if somewhere there wasn't an office pool swelling with bets on whether or not these broken people would go through with the adoption. In restaurants all over town, good friends of theirs and mere acquaintances exchanged judgments over lunch. "It's too soon." "They're going to regret it." "It's too soon." "They've forgotten what it's like to have a baby in the house." "Andy will freak out." "They're too old." "They're too shattered."

"They're too desperate." "They're trying to replace Emily ... don't they know they can't do that?" "It's too soon."

I know how the conversations went, because as embarrassing as it is to admit, I sometimes participated. On some days I too passed judgment, not out of cattiness or mean-spiritedness, but out of worry for my dear friends' well-being. On other days I applauded their decision as though they had just resolved to separate the land from the sea, the light from the darkness, and create the world.

I've never lost a child. I don't let the thought of that possibility enter my consciousness. I certainly don't know how I would mourn. I don't know how hard is hard enough or how long is long enough, and I don't think I would care. I don't know why any of us thought we knew how to mourn better than Emily's parents did.

A month after Sara's adoption, her new parents and brother held a baby-naming ceremony at their synagogue. After an apocalyptic year, we watched them smile for the first time. It wasn't the proud, youthful, confident smile they radiated at Emily. This was a new smile for Sara. It had love in it and also fear. It was a wise and world-weary smile. It was the most courageous smile I had ever seen.

In their bones, these parents understand that Sara has not come to them to replace Emily, but to glorify her. The experience of parenting their daughter was so profound, they couldn't bear to face the years ahead without it. Only the greatest of loves empowers us with the valor it takes to love again despite the risk.

Sara's Chinese birth mother must have loved her too, so deeply that she abandoned her in a place where she knew the child would be found and cared for. I've imagined her, hiding in the night, soaked with tears, holding a private vigil until her daughter, her soul mate, was carried away to safety. I believe she dreams today that her daughter will be raised in a land where little girls are as precious as their brothers—where little girls can be dancers *and* doctors. Two broken women a world apart have been inextricably linked through their grief. Their losses are allowing a new child to dream.

The three townships have stopped whispering now. They long ago moved on to gossip about a forty-year-old woman who recently lost her husband to cancer. Word has it that she has accepted a dinner invitation from a man. I don't think it's too soon to order dessert.

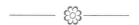

Karin Kasdin is an award-winning author and playwright. Her most recent book is *Watsammata U: A Get-a-Grip Guide to Staying Sane Through Your Child's College Application Process.* She is the mother of three sons. Emily was Karin's beloved drama student, baby-sitter, and, along with the rest of her family members, Jim, JoAnn, Andy, and Sara, a very special friend. Sara is flourishing in her new family.

It Doesn't Keep Me from Smiling

Latoya Chivon Maddox

My name is Latoya Chivon Maddox, and I am going to tell you about my life and why I think of it as half full. On October 19, 1983, I entered the world at the University of Pennsylvania. I was born with athrogryposis, a disability that keeps most of the joints in my body locked, with the exception of my neck and shoulders. That means I basically have no use of my arms or legs. I am typing this at a computer with a pencil in my mouth. With a pencil, I can turn on the computer and log on, and then I can write just like you. My teachers and classmates tell me that I have the neatest handwriting of anyone in my school!

My aide's name is Kathy Clark, and she's been with me since fifth grade. She is my arms and legs during school hours. It's like having your mother go to school with you, but I've been in foster care since I was a little kid, so sometimes it is nice to have a motherly figure around.

A lot of people choose to focus on what I can't do. Okay, I can't run or tie my shoes or feed myself or give someone a hug. But I'd rather think about what I can do. Even though my legs and arms don't move, my right elbow has enough motion to let me operate my motorized wheelchair so I can blast down the hallways at school. I can paint, and draw cartoons, and turn pages, and use this computer. Most important, I can still smile.

If you heard about what happened to me when I was a baby, you'd think maybe I shouldn't be smiling so much. But ask my friends. I giggle a lot, and I do have a lot of friends. I sing in the choir. I wore a pretty lilac, strapless dress to the prom. Why would I want to go to the prom, if I can't dance? You should see the way I can move my head and shoulders!

I got my first electric wheelchair when I was about four or five, and I'll never forget it. I was going down the hallway at Widener Memorial School asking my physical therapist, How do I stop the chair? She told me just to let the joystick go. *Slam.* I crashed into the library door. I guess I should have taken my hand off the joystick. But I'm not going to live in fear. My hand's been on that joystick ever since.

I'm a regular student, at a regular public school—Neshamany High School in Pennsylvania—but I guess no one would say I've had a regular life. I lived with my mother, father, and my brothers and sister until I was six. I got put into foster care a month and a half before my sixth birthday, not knowing that my life would probably never be the same again. It was a Friday morning, and my mother had just returned from walking my older sister and brother to the door so that they could go to school. She said her stomach was hurting, then I heard a splash. Her waters had broken. She took me and my brother, Reggie, down to the kitchen and told us to stay there, and she would be right back. I didn't see her for almost two years.

My first foster home was nice, but I could not face the fact that social services took us all away from each other. I had some nice foster homes with some people who took good care of me, and some foster homes that I really don't want to talk about, so let's move on. But all I wanted was for my mother to come get me to take me home so that we could be one big family again.

I was lucky enough to have a social worker, Ms. Ann, who always came to my rescue. She would come for a visit and take me home with her. She would cook me my favorite meal—spaghetti—and let me sit on the counter next to her. Then one day, in a family counseling session, who should come strolling through the door but my mother. My heart, well, you could either say it jumped out of my chest or the bottom of my stomach, I was so excited to see her.

But living with my mom again wasn't meant to be. My fantasy was just too good to be true. My mother was still sick. She said that when she was better she would be able to take care of us.

In 1993, I moved into a group home for disabled children, Wood Services. My first full day there was pretty exciting. One of the staff asked me, since I couldn't go to school until I'd had all my shots, if I wanted to go to the mall with her. Sure I did! She bought me my first pair of earrings with my birthstone in them. I was so happy. Then as we were leaving the mall, a man walked up to me and handed me a twenty-dollar bill. I couldn't reach out and take it from him, and I'm thinking, what's this for? The staff person told me that no one could resist my smile.

When I was young, the kids would tease me because I couldn't walk or use my hands. My father would tell me, "Don't be afraid—you are what you are." One day, when I was four or five years old, a boy was teasing me, and my sister was warning him that he better leave me alone. He didn't believe her, and sure enough, I got him. I'm not going to say what I did, but he never bothered me again.

I still live at the group home, but now I attend regular high school. I'm going to graduate this year. I'm eighteen, and I plan to go to college next year. I will soon be moving to another group home where I hope to grow socially and get the care that I need. I am now in touch with my mother, who has a job now and is doing much better. She is trying to get a house so that me, my sister, and my little brothers can live with her again.

Sometimes I become totally depressed and stressed out over my disability. I need help going to the bathroom, taking a shower, and getting dressed. But then I realize that if I don't let people help me, how will these things get done?

When I'm feeling down, I remind myself: "I know God made us all different for a reason." I often ask myself, "Why me?" Hopefully some day I will find out.

When I graduate from college, I want to be a prosecutor, a career I've wanted for myself ever since watching courtroom shows on television. A winning smile can't hurt me in the courtroom, wouldn't you say?

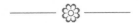

Latoya wrote this story to open the minds of other disabled children and let them have a better understanding that "life is what you make it." Latoya hopes that in the near and distant future she will keep on becoming the best that she can be, and that she will overcome any new obstacles on her path.

Fried-Egg Sandwiches

Liesel Shineberg

*A*s a young child, I didn't always know that the misery I was experiencing had a so-called silver lining, or that, as an adult, I would grow up to admire the very people whom I once so feared or held in awe from a distance. One incident remains firm in my memory, of a teacher who I now understand was one of the most remarkable people I've ever known.

My cousin, Werner, and I lived with our aunt Frieda Reiss in 1939 while our parents still resided in the camp for refugees in Rotterdam, which the Dutch government had opened to house thousands of Jews who were crossing the border.

My aunt engaged the services of a teacher to help Werner and me learn the rudiments of English. Her name was Juffrouw Meyers. We came to her home one afternoon a week after our regular school in Amsterdam. She sat so close to the electric heater that I always worried that her skirt would catch fire. She had a perpetual cold and, evidently, only one handkerchief, which she would wave over the stove to dry each time she blew her nose.

She was short, plump, and homely. Her face was deeply lined, and her double chin hung in folds. Age marks covered her cheeks, but I rather admired her nose, which was high and, I thought, patrician looking. She was in her late seventies. She always wore the same long black skirt and a long-sleeved blouse of an unidentifiable color with tattered lace.

Her apartment in a tall, gray building in Amsterdam was always cold, the furnishings shabby and drab. There was always a mixed odor of cabbage, laundry, and camphor. It was January, and winters in Holland were chilly and damp. Our shoes would often adhere to the ice, so we would wrap our shoes with rags. By the time we got to our destination the rags would have worn off, so we'd have to walk carefully so our leather soles would not stick and get ruined.

Juffrouw Meyers had the quavering voice of an old person, but it still was strong enough to scold us when our accent offended her. She took the money which Aunt Frieda gave us to pay for our lessons with quick fingers, and the bills immediately disappeared into the side pocket of her skirt.

"Remember, in America they will respect you if you speak their language" was her refrain as she kept after us. "Study!" That was the main message.

We studied with her for six months and learned basic English conversation. It took us a while to pick up the vernacular. I distinctly remember a popular song with the line, "Jim never sends me pretty flowers." For the longest time I could not figure out what gym, a class I took in school, had to do with pretty flowers. The years passed, and occasionally I thought of my teacher. I realized later that she gave sanctuary to refugees with no place to go. The money from our lessons undoubtedly helped to feed the hordes and the smell probably was cabbage, which was inexpensive. Most likely she could not afford to heat the apartment, and the stove was turned on only during the times she gave lessons. Holland did not have a welfare program for refugees in those days, and it must have been a struggle to survive.

I realize now that she was truly a decent and caring human being. I wonder about what happened to her. She was old, after all, and with the country under German control, she would have been among the first to be deported.

"Remember," she would say to Werner and me, sitting in her wooden chair. "Remember!"

I am remembering her. Thinking about her, I recall another kind soul that I met when our family finally came to the United States in 1940. How one person can make a difference, can turn darkness into light. I hope, by some remarkable coincidence, that this woman with whom I am no longer in touch will come across this book, read my story about her, and know how she positively changed my life, much as my teacher, Juffrouw Meyers, did.

My family lived in a fifth-floor tenement building in New York. It wasn't really a walk-up, since it did have an elevator, but the attendant stuck out his hand for a tip each time one entered and, only having money for bare necessities, we walked up.

My father took me to the nearest grade school, located on Nicholas Avenue, near 150th Street. We opened the gate and stepped into the schoolyard. The majority of the students were black. I was not prepared for this, since I had not been in the presence of black people before. I have often wondered if a black child, suddenly thrust into a white world, feels the same insecurity.

The students and teachers worked with me and, among the multitude, I found a handful of other students, refugees like myself, who helped me to understand English, which I found to be quite confusing. Mother found a job as a maid, and Dad peddled sugared almonds, which we made at night in our kitchen and packed into cellophane bags, up and down Broadway.

Money was really scarce—we ate very simply. Mother would pack a small slice of dry bread for my lunch. I found a water fountain and that made it go down easier.

One day, Sydonia, a black girl with a head full of little braids and long skinny legs, who sat at the next desk, said to me, "My Momma said that you have to come home with me for supper today." She probably saw that I did not have anywhere to go for the midday meal and watched me eat my slice of bread. I was shocked! Was this an order? What was this word, *supper*? I was so intimidated that I let her lead me to her home at noon.

A large, kind-faced lady with a big smile opened the door. She wore a blue dress with a large, multicolored apron tied around her ample middle, and she pulled me through the door giving me a big hug. It was Sydonia's mother. They lived in an apartment much like mine, poorly furnished, but clean with wonderful odors of something cooking.

"You poor child. My Sydonia says you are hungry. Well, you sit down and eat!"

A plate with a fried-egg sandwich and a glass of milk was put in front of me. I had never seen a sandwich like this. "Eat, while it is hot," the mother ordered. I did not need a second invitation. It was delicious! I remembered my good manners before we went back to school, thanked her to the best of my English-speaking ability, and stuck out my hand. She grabbed it, pulled me to her, and gave me another hug.

"You come back now," she said.

I could not wait for Mother to come home from work that evening so I could tell her about my adventure. My mother was born into wealth but had to leave everything behind in a country that no longer wanted her. She and Daddy had to start from scratch to help make a new life for themselves and their family. And here, in another country, a stranger, probably in the same financial condition that we were in, was feeding her child. She was overcome with regret for not being able to do more for me, admiration for

Sydonia's mother, and shame, perhaps because she probably would not have done the same for a black child.

The next day Mom took her pride in hand and enrolled me in the free school lunch program. But only for a while, until she and Dad got their feet on the ground. Then I took a proper sandwich with me and, occasionally, an extra treat for Sydonia.

As my language skills improved, I often thought about Juffrouw Meyers and hoped that she would have been proud of me. Now, when my grandsons pile into our house after school, starving, they say (of course, they will never know *starving* the way that I knew it), I always fix them a quick fried-egg sandwich.

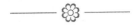

Liesel is a naturalized proud American citizen, born in Aachen, Germany, now living in Rock Springs, Wyoming, with her husband, Edward. They are both actively retired with two wonderful daughters, two granddaughters, and two grandsons. Liesel travels the state keeping the memories of the Holocaust alive for a younger generation. Every day she is grateful for special people like Juffrouw Meyers and Sydonia's mom, who helped her survive difficult times.

Johnny

Lorrell Holtz-Oxley

Optimism is not necessarily my strongest suit. After fifteen-plus years in the career world, I've gotten pretty cynical. In 1995, I took a bold step and left a good job to start my own consulting business. I thought I was doing this for my career and my psyche. But maybe I was doing it for Johnny, and I did not even know it.

What I might lack in natural optimism is balanced by a very high level of perseverance. I am "TSTQ"—Too Stupid to Quit. I have succeeded in many arenas simply because I worked harder than anyone else. However, I nearly met my match earlier this year—in Johnny.

Three years ago I had a husband and a career, and no children, by choice. That was before the house across the street burned down. One doesn't think of a house fire as a "block party," but the fire brought all of us together as we gawked at the blaze. In the midst of the crowd a little boy, just seven years old, was showing his gregarious nature by striking up conversations with neighbors assembled for this event. This was the first time I met Johnny, who lived down the street.

The next day Johnny rang our doorbell. He was just coming for a visit. I was surprised but let him in. Admittedly, I was more annoyed than anything at the interruption. The next day it happened again, and then the day after that, and on and on. Soon he was spending a significant amount of time with us. Honestly, my husband and I were perturbed about this turn of events. His visits were getting in the way of my consulting assignments and were consuming significant amounts of time. Where was his mother during all the time he was at our home? I was feeling quite judgmental of her.

As the weeks went by, we learned that Johnny lived with his mother and two teenage sisters in a home with an absent father who has been frequently incarcerated and has never paid a dime in child support. Johnny's mother worked several jobs to barely keep their family's heads above water. Johnny was lonely, unruly, and often angry. He had plenty of reason to be.

And there was something else that infuriated this kind-hearted and very intelligent boy: he couldn't read.

His keen memory, highly observant nature, and a strong ability to fake it helped him hide his problem until we noticed that he never laughed at funny signs or words in cartoons. Now that Johnny was at our home four or five hours a day during the week and all day long on weekends, we felt called to help.

We bought various types of reading software. He ignored it or exploded in self-hatred and desperation when he didn't understand the words, which was often. By this time he was headed to fourth grade but struggling greatly with first-grade-level books.

We decided that I would forego consulting assignments for the summer in order to focus on helping Johnny improve his reading level. We worked out a system of rewards for reading things out loud—candy, small toys, a trip for pizza or the roller rink—things that were very motivational to a child with few possessions.

Although Johnny did, encouragingly, improve a grade level within three months, he had severe reading problems I couldn't fix and the telltale signs of dyslexia. Every reading session was long and stressful. I yearned for the days when I had been in control of my life and sure of myself. Each day seemed to present a greater struggle than the one before. Beyond all that, we had wanted to move out of the neighborhood into a larger house. Now it seemed we were tied to this neighborhood, and to this little boy, for years to come.

The public schools were of little or no help. We attended the parent-teacher conferences along with his mother, and despite Johnny's high level of intelligence, we were merely encouraged to lower our expectations. Aghast at the school's various responses to our requests, and desperate for help, I researched reading disabilities on the Internet. There I discovered Currey Ingram Academy School, an innovative college preparatory school right under my nose here in Nashville, which specializes in children who have average to superior IQs and learning differences.

Its campus, in a ritzy part of town, seemed perfect for Johnny. They used all the proven methods for teaching dyslexics that I couldn't get the school system to consider, and a record of success that included children who have been accepted at Harvard. I toured the facilities and was amazed at what I saw.

Then I saw the numbers for tuition. Including uniforms, books, school trips, and the like, it would run about twenty grand a year. My heart sank. I could buy a nice car for the amount of money they required in yearly tuition. A *very* nice car. And Johnny would need years at that school. The school was totally out of our financial reach, and certainly of his mother's.

My questions about financial aid at introductory meetings about the school were met with somewhat icy responses. We were told that parents could write off the tuition on their taxes if a doctor prescribed the school for their child. I sighed. This mother doesn't have the money to send him, so writing off the tuition won't help her a bit. And besides, Johnny's mom hadn't even set foot in my home in the entire three years we'd known him. How would I persuade her to fill out the very extensive application form and financial aid report?

Once excited, I was now more chagrined than ever. All my effort and work seemed pointless. Refusing to give up, though, because of my TSTQ nature, I started doing more research. I left a message with the regional dyslexia association hot line and the next day, a dyslexia expert at a local university returned the call.

I briefly explained Johnny's situation, and she said, "You really shouldn't give up hope on Currey Ingram. I know some children there right now on full scholarships." I hadn't mentioned Currey Ingram at all. We hadn't even discussed schools. Why did she bring it up at all? It was spooky. But the message was not lost on me. I was sure this was a "dope slap from God."

We called Johnny's mother, and unbelievably, she agreed to meet with us the next day. She spent several hours at our home watching a video about the school and learning more about their programs. She agreed that we needed to go through the time-consuming process of making every attempt to get Johnny into the school, and she completed the very complicated and long financial aid forms. She attended school tours with me. This was a very significant change. Perhaps God had given us both a little hope that we desperately needed.

I bought law books about statutes regarding learning disabilities. I got Johnny tested. I went to conferences on dyslexia. I made myself visible (but not obnoxious) at Currey Ingram Academy.

The day came for Johnny's visit to Currey Ingram. It was designed as a "tryout" to see how he fit in with the rest of the students and to do some additional testing. Partway through the day I got a call from Johnny's mother. The director of admissions had called her to tell her how wonderfully he was fitting in. She said no one had ever gotten so many positive comments from teachers regarding their manners and sociability. Our testing results were "dead on," and she said, "if ever a child needed to be here, it's Johnny."

Johnny enjoyed his visit greatly. After he left, he said, "I really think God is going to get me into Currey Ingram. He has done so many good things for me already, why would he stop now?"

I smiled and cried inside at his comment. "Honey, I hope you're right," I said. "But if not, we have some other good options lined up." I knew that every other alternative paled in comparison. I was afraid for him to get his hopes up.

Every week of waiting was torture. I doubted far more than I believed. One day I went to lunch with my husband at a Chinese restaurant. My fortune read, "Your hard work will soon pay off." I don't put much stock in fortunes, but this time I knew God was giving me a message I needed.

When we returned home, a message awaited us. Currey Ingram was making a place for Johnny at their school on a full scholarship. I wept with joy and great relief, and Johnny was ecstatic. Just knowing that he was assured of attending that school produced a change in his disposition that was amazing.

There are still so many struggles for this little boy and his family—such daunting ones that I recognize my lack of resources to handle them. Through this experience, though, I have come to appreciate the resources I do have, and I have learned anew what it means to depend on God, and to give it another try when I would much rather quit entirely.

Johnny was an "inconvenient change in my agenda." But God knew what Johnny and I needed before we did. When my husband and I "decided" not to have children, God was laughing.

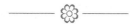

Lorrell Holtz-Oxley is a consultant to call centers and music companies and owner of a candle-making business. She lives in Nashville, Tennessee, with her husband, David, a computer engineer, and three cats. They have no children of their own, but you'd never know that if you stopped by their home after school. Several children from homes with their own sets of challenges now hang out at the Holtz-Oxleys. Johnny, now eleven, is enrolled at Currey Ingram Academy, where he plans on joining the chess club. He wants to be a lawyer, inventor, mathematician, or engineer when he grows up.

I Never Knew
Who I Would Be

Mary Emma Allen

"*H*ow awful that your mother had Alzheimer's. It's such a terrible disease. How did you ever survive?" I'm frequently asked.

Years ago, if someone had predicted I'd care for Mother during her journey through Alzheimer's after Father's death, I'd never have believed them. Nor would I have imagined Mother allowing this. She had been a very independent lady throughout the years, wanting control over her life.

All I'd heard were horror stories about Alzheimer's when I first realized Mother might be following the path her sister trod. Although Auntie also had Alzheimer's, I had only intermittent contact with her and wasn't responsible for her day-to-care care. Yes, there were frustrations, disappointments, and bittersweet memories as Mother and I struggled to adjust to this situation, first in her home, then in mine, and eventually in a nursing home when she required more care than I could give. Sometimes she was obstinate and probably thought I was, since I insisted, for her safety, that she follow my instructions.

When I wouldn't let her stay alone because she wandered in the snow half dressed, she remarked, "If you went out to the clothesline in your bathrobe and slippers, no one would get a sitter for you."

Our role reversal, as I became the parent to my parent, was fraught with frustrations. Then talking with my neighbor, who had cared for a great-aunt with Alzheimer's, reading all I could to understand this disease that was capturing my mother, and attending workshops helped me look at the situation from Mother's view and develop an understanding of her.

The fact that she often couldn't remember who I was brought interesting situations into our lives. I never knew who I might be when I awoke in the morning while she lived with me. It's a shock at first to realize your own mother doesn't know you. However, I couldn't change the situation, couldn't force her to remember. So why not be another person for the day and enjoy the adventure?

Sometimes Mother thought I was her older sister, perhaps because I was now in the role of caregiver as her sister had been when they were growing up on a farm. Fortunately, because I'd heard Mother's stories throughout my life, I knew enough about the people in her past to carry on those conversations from another era. My being

"Auntie" gave Mother pleasure. It only confused her if I tried to correct her and thus take her sister away.

Most interesting were those occasions when I became "that other woman" in mother's mind. She would at times become convinced that I was not her daughter, married to her son-in-law, but "another woman" who was trying to steal her daughter's husband away. I turned into this home wrecker at the most unexpected times, and Mother tried to chase me away. The next morning she might tell me, "She was here last night. But I didn't let her stay."

I discovered the saving grace a sense of humor brings when caring for a person afflicted with Alzheimer's. Instead of scolding Mother about something she couldn't remember two minutes later, I learned to laugh with her. When my husband and I found Mother's imaginary chickens amusing, she looked at us, puzzled, then commented, "We don't laugh enough." A smile enveloped her face. I realized Mother needed more laughter in her life, and I did too.

Gradually, I learned to enjoy the small rewards. To see a smile appear when I patted her cheek, to watch her face brighten at the sound of my voice, to have her reach out to hold my hand when I sat beside her chair ... these joys outweighed the times she didn't know me or gave me a difficult time.

As Mother became more childlike, we still experienced good times together. I visited her in her world and gained insight into her thoughts and condition. We listened to music together, talked of days gone by, had tea parties, and picked flowers in the garden outside her room at the nursing home. Small pleasures excited Mother even more than they once did and caused me to stop and enjoy the wonder of the world again.

Alzheimer's gradually brought a gentleness to Mother that endeared her to the staff at the nursing home and surprised her family, who was accustomed to a domineering woman. In a lucid moment, she might ask me a question about the family business my father left. But then confusion would overtake her and she'd say, "You're taking care of it, aren't you?" Eventually she stopped asking or insisting I do it her way.

Sometimes Alzheimer's is a blessing in disguise to the victims as they escape from life's problems and responsibilities. This especially proved true when my brother committed suicide. At first Mother was cognizant of his death. However, eventually the disease brought blessed forgetfulness. It kept Mother in a world where my brother still lived, and it protected her from the devastating grief she would have known otherwise.

Even though I struggled with placing my mother in a nursing home, she adjusted to this environment more readily than we had imagined. Perhaps it helped that I had used the nursing home for day care before Mother became a full-time resident. Once there, she created her own world within the home, often thinking she was back on the farm of her girlhood.

Family ties gave meaning to Mother's days even when she was in her own world. I watched my daughter and grandchildren interact with her and knew they brought Mother pleasure while they learned the joy of serving others. Their visits were the high points of her days, even though she might not know who they were. The children accepted this and learned to enjoy giving her pleasure.

"Such good children," she remarked one day as Kara and Alex sat near her chair and drew pictures. Another time she watched them, with a group of children, gathering Easter eggs during a hunt at the nursing home. As she laughed with the youngsters, I wondered if she was remembering her days of teaching in a one-room school.

Loving Mother and caring for her throughout this disease, though laced with sadness and frustration, eventually brought a new dimension to my love for her. In a world where I couldn't alter Mother's condition, I learned God's lesson of giving pleasure, with its unexpected rewards ... a deeper love and appreciation of this lady who once had cared for me.

Mary Emma's mother died in January 2001, after being afflicted with Alzheimer's for more than twelve years. Mary Emma is glad she and her family could be there for her. Mary Emma Allen writes for children and adults. Many of her pieces appear in inspirational publications like *Heartwarmers of Spirit*. Her book, *When We Become the Parent of Our Parents*, describes her mother's journey through Alzheimer's.

A God-Given Confidence

Nancy B. Gibbs

"Nobody would ever believe how shy you were when I met you," my husband, Roy, whispered. He hugged me as I stepped down from behind the podium.

I had just stood before our church and presented an inspirational message for the annual Woman's Day service. I wasn't at all shaky or nervous. I had all the confidence in the world. I haven't always been able to speak before a crowd, however. As a matter of fact, if I was in a room with more than two people, I kept quiet and simply listened to what everyone else had to say.

When I was a child, I had very little confidence in myself. I was very timid. I only had a few friends at school. It wasn't that the other students disliked me; they just didn't know me. I didn't play, laugh, or talk with them. Although I had one close friend, I pretty much kept to myself. I didn't enjoy school, nor did I much like myself. I was very lonely as I lived in my quiet and reserved world.

A nine-week speech class was mandatory in high school. I panicked when I stood in front of the class and attempted to recite a poem. I could barely speak. When I finally forced the words out, I forgot most of the stanzas. When I ran back to my desk, tears of embarrassment filled my eyes.

"I'm never speaking in front of a group of people again," I vowed.

Quite a few years later, I married the man of my dreams. My husband, Roy, is a minister. Speaking before a crowd is easy for him. I envied him. To me, some of the most difficult days of our newly married life were the times we were being introduced at new churches. I very seldom spoke. I simply stood there staring at the floor, praying that nobody would ask me a question.

As a hobby, I signed up for a ceramics class at the local recreation center. I enjoyed the class and worked hard on my projects, but like before, I only listened while the other students talked and laughed. One day, Roy met a fellow student of mine. I was ashamed when he told me that she had mentioned how quiet I was. It was at that moment that I knew I had to change, even though I didn't have any clue how.

I prayed that God would change me from the inside out. I begged Him to give me a boost of confidence. Somehow He gave me the strength I needed. I took a leap of faith, because I knew that I had to go way out of my comfort zone and try something that I had always deemed impossible. I took a sales position that required me to stand before several women to demonstrate a product that I was selling.

As I drove to the very first presentation, I prayed. I turned around and headed back home three times before I finally found myself in the parking lot in front of the hostess's apartment.

"I can't believe I'm doing this, God," I prayed. "Please be with me." I got out of the car, went inside, and was greeted by a dozen smiling ladies. I began to perspire and tremble.

"With God's help, I can do this," I reassured myself.

To my great relief, the ladies were receptive to me, and I closed several sales. I booked three additional presentations and was on my way to a successful career. I could feel it down deep in my soul. All the way home I thanked God for His graciousness.

A few weeks passed, and several times I became the top salesperson of the week for this company. I won some nice prizes and awards. More important, however, I discovered that I could do anything that I wanted to do, if I allowed God to work through me.

Roy was both happy about and surprised at the changes I made in my life. While we were always able to discuss his goals and dreams, he was concerned that I didn't talk about what I wanted to do with my life. I realized that the lack of confidence that I held kept me from dreaming. Now we share mutual dreams as we work together in our church—he as the pastor and me as the senior lady's Sunday school teacher and mission director.

God worked a great miracle in my life when he turned my shyness into confidence. In gratitude, whenever possible, I accept all invitations to speak of God's greatness. I often think that my shyness must have been part of God's great plan. If I had been born with the gift to speak from childhood, I would never have realized that my speaking ability is a direct gift from God. What I thought of all those years as my "curse" of shyness turned out to be part of God's plan.

This time, when I cry after speaking to a crowd, I'm not crying the unhappy tears that filled my eyes during that speech class some thirty years earlier. These are happy tears, the kind that God loves to see.

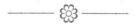

Nancy lives in South Georgia with her husband and pastor, Roy. They serve together at a small church. Nancy writes a weekly religion column. She enjoys speaking at women's mission groups in her community. She is very proud of her accomplishments since she escaped the insecure feelings that once held her back. Nancy feels that her greatest accomplishments lie in her grown children, Brad, Chad, and Becky and her precious granddaughter, Hannah.

Lost in a Big City

Nanci Stroupe

God enjoys helping us, even in small ways. One day my daughter, who was about twelve at the time, and I took off for Richmond, Virginia, to watch her daddy play in a fast pitch softball tournament. My husband had awakened me earlier to go with him, but I was still sleepy and assured him I would have no trouble finding it by myself and if I had a problem, I certainly had a mouth to ask for directions if I needed to.

Well, Hubby really didn't think I would attempt to find him in Richmond because there is a lot of traffic there and it's a big place a couple of hours away. The only directions he gave me was that the ballpark was located behind a 7-Eleven store and that it was near a park of some kind. When Lisa and I woke up, we jumped in the car and headed out from our home for what we thought would be a two-hour drive at most.

Little did we know—there must be hundreds of 7-Eleven stores in Richmond, and I didn't know the name of the park. Lisa and I both had an adventurous spirit so we drove and drove, searching for the ball game.

We stumbled into a town lost in time. Cars were parked along the main street, pulled in toward the curb, not parallel parked, which seemed strange to me. Everyone was out shopping, this being a Saturday, and this busy little town had a very sweet sense of security in the air. I had been driving now for almost four hours and was thinking perhaps I'd better head back home, if I could figure out where home was.

We spotted a policeman and asked for his help. We explained our predicament to him, and he was very kind and offered to help us find my husband. He proceeded to get on his radio and said to follow him. Lisa thought it was very cool to have a policeman leading the way with flashing lights. If we were very lucky, we would find her daddy and catch an inning or two of the last game. Off we went with the lights flashing.

We went from ballpark to ballpark, with the policeman radioing his police buddies to try to help us. When we had tried all the ballparks around or near a 7-Eleven store in Richmond, he was about to give up when he remembered one more. At this point, I was pretty sure Lisa and I would be heading back home very soon, tired and disappointed.

We really believe in the power of prayer, and so we prayed some more, and this time God answered our prayers. The policeman led us into the last park he could think of, and I recognized my husband's car. Dad's game was in progress, and they all stopped for a moment when they heard the sirens. We thanked the policeman over and over and started walking down the first-base line.

Doug was pitching and I started hollering, "Fire it in there, Dougie, throw that ball hard!" At this point he was in his fifth game of the day and it was ninety-eight degrees. He was exhausted, but when he heard Lisa and me hollering, he got his second wind, started firing that ball, and he retired the side.

Dougie won the tournament that day by pitching five consecutive games in the heat. Later, as we laughed about my strange adventure and I told him about how Lisa had spotted our guardian angel, the policeman, in that strange little town, we knew we could search the whole of Richmond over again and we'd never find that quaint little town again.

I learned a very valuable lesson that day. God was right there with us all the time, just waiting for us to ask for help. When we did, God responded. Now I don't wait so long before I ask God for help. I know God will lead me in the right direction, whether it's through a problem in life or through a street in a big city.

My husband might have won the tournament that day, but I got an even better reward when Lisa and I went searching for his game: unbreakable faith in God.

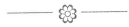

Nanci Stroupe is a writer with stories published in *Heartwarmers of Love and Courage* and *Stories for a Woman's Heart*. She lives in Hampton, Virginia, very happily with her husband, Doug, who is retired from NASA and plays golf every day that ends with a Y. While Doug is golfing, Nanci is either having lunch with her friends or working on another story. She loves writing about her childhood and all the funny things that happened to her. They also enjoy spending time with their daughter Sherry and her son, Dusty, their daughter Lisa and her husband, Mike, and their granddaughters, Ashley, Emily, Anastasia, Amber, and Angelina.

Heightened Senses

Patty Mooney

I knew the concept intellectually, that enlightenment can often come when you are the most terrified. Little did I know that one Saturday this last April I would feel the truth of this statement in my gut. And that I would be grateful for the experience!

My husband, five male friends, and I gathered at a trailhead forty miles from Palm Springs in anticipation of our annual mountain-bike ride in the high desert that finishes in Palm Springs.

We do this trek once a year, right after the daylight savings time shift, because it is what we call a "death march," and we need that extra hour of daylight. Barring any unforeseen technical difficulties, the ride takes at least seven hours. The wilderness there is so gorgeous, and our annual ritual so dear to us, we felt compelled to ride, even under the threat of hundred-degree weather.

That morning, to check out my gears, I pedaled down the road away from the group about an eighth of a mile. I had a sudden urge to relieve my bladder. Just as I set my bike down and stepped toward a bush, I heard what sounded like the roar of an engine. My second almost immediate thought was, "What engine? There are no cars here!" As my heart beat wildly and a sudden perspiration rose all over my body, I jumped back on my bike in a panic and sped back to the trailhead.

I knew that noise had come from a lion, and I had been too close to be safe. When I told the boys about my animal encounter, they all leaped aboard their bikes and rode down to the area. I followed them, my courage bolstered by being surrounded by six men, to show them exactly where I'd heard the roar.

My husband, Mark, walked behind the bush and found mountain-lion prints about ten feet from where I'd been. "Looks like it had to be at least a hundred pounds," Mark said. I was thrilled about the paw prints because it meant that I had not been hearing things. It validated my experience. I also felt somehow special that I had encountered such an extraordinary animal.

Soon it was time to start riding. About five miles downhill, my rear rim hit some sharp rocks and split, which meant that I would not be able to continue the ride (we had thirty-five more miles to go). My heart sank; I had been looking forward to this ride for a long time. But I could see that there would be no way to jury-rig the bike, and that was that. The guys were actually more upset than I was, which touched me.

I told them that I would walk the bike back up to the trailhead. They all looked at each other; I could tell they were wondering who would "draw the short straw" in riding back with me. As the ride leader (the person who knows the trail), Mark would have to continue on. I knew that nobody wanted to drop out of this long-anticipated ride.

"I'll go alone," I said, "It's simple. I'll just follow our tire tracks." Mark asked Wes to give me his keys (his truck was parked at a campground four miles from the trail-head), and David handed me his cell phone.

Mark looked into my eyes and asked, "Are you okay with this?" I reassured him that I was fine. Truthfully, a part of me wanted him to come to my rescue and escort me up the mountain; I was acting braver than I was really feeling. But I didn't want to deprive him of an experience he had been wanting as badly as I had. We hugged and parted ways, promising to catch up at the end of the day.

The thought of a stalking mountain lion followed me practically every minute of my uphill trek. "He could be watching me, and I would never know it." I thought, "Maybe he can see that I am a female of the species and thus easier to catch." "How much more obvious can I be in my red Lycra outfit?" This is when I learned about the gift of fear.

For my hyperawareness of the possible presence of this lion was an extraordinary gift. That uphill trek, although not what I had initially wanted for myself at all, was the most intense and monumental experience I have ever had in the desert, before or since. It was like having my third eye peeled open. All my senses were sharp, and I saw the beauty around me in a whole new light.

Instead of turning into a snarling, resentful bitch, cursing my technical breakdown, which had made me miss out on an epic ride, or having one big pity-party about being abandoned by all my friends and having to trudge up five unending miles in dangerous heat, I totally bypassed this woe-is-me place, which in the past has only resulted in bags under my eyes and a less than stellar attitude.

Because of my momentary encounter with the lion, I couldn't have planned a more engaging and spiritual journey! When I spotted the road, I was almost disappointed that my journey was nearly at an end. Even relating it now brings me back there, as I feel a hot breeze on my neck, and I see blackened ocotillo against an impossibly blue sky.

What could have been just an ordeal was transformed into paradise, thanks to a mountain lion's appearance and just enough fear to fully awaken my senses.

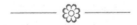

Patty Mooney practices her arts in San Diego, where she and her husband are partners at New & Unique Videos, a stock footage library, and Crystal Pyramid Productions, a broadcast video production company.

No More Fear

Penny Frost

The argument with Robert was the last straw. We had just had our fourth child three months before, and we were still fighting. I had to take a walk to cool off. Thoughts of life with Robert were running through my mind as I briskly tramped the dark streets of Lewiston.

My feet were getting tired. I stopped into a dance club on Lisbon Street to get a drink and some much-needed rest. I sat down at a small empty table and slipped my shoes off beneath it. A handsome man with a very kind face brought me a drink.

"A frown is very unbecoming on such a beautiful face. Is this seat taken?" he asked as he slid into the seat in front of me.

"No. Knock yourself out," I answered.

His name was Bruce (not his real name). Before long, he had me dancing and laughing. I found him very kind, caring, funny, and easy to talk to. He let me ramble on about my troubled marriage while he listened intently, never once offering advice or opinions, just listening. I felt like a princess, a feeling I've never had before. When the club was getting ready to close, I thought for sure that this time I had found my Prince Charming.

I waited until morning to tell Robert I was going to file for divorce as soon as the courthouse opened. Robert understood and was actually relieved. We had been arguing, it seemed, since the day we got married. Robert arranged to have his things picked up later that evening.

The following morning, I opened the door to get the newspaper, and there were a dozen red roses, lying at my feet. Inside the card was a dinner invitation and a note that read, "Yours always, Bruce."

Bruce seemed to have an endless supply of cash. The next few weeks were filled with dinners, dancing, flowers, expensive wines, and foliage trips. I began to feel guilty and wondered if I was going to break the man. When I asked him about his money situation, he laughed and took me for a drive. Out in the middle of a huge sandpit were several trucks with his last name on every one of them. Bruce was a contractor. My mind was finally at ease, and once again, I was enjoying my wonderful fairy-tale romance. I was filled with optimism about the future.

Bruce found us a beautiful three-bedroom house on the lake. The view was breathtaking. We often went shopping so that I could furnish the house any way I wanted. Nothing was too expensive for Bruce.

"Buy whatever you want. After all, you're the one who will be spending the most time there," Bruce said.

Little did I know how very true those words would become.

Maybe I should have seen it coming, but there were no warning signs that I recognized. We had been living together a short while when one day Bruce came home in a bad mood. He was obviously very disturbed about something. He called the sitter, then informed me that we were going for a ride. I had never seen him in such a foul mood. We patiently waited for the sitter to arrive, then we got into the truck. Bruce spun out of the driveway and proceeded to drive at a very alarming speed. I begged him to slow down and tell me what was wrong. In the same instant, he slammed on the brakes. My head slammed into the windshield so hard that it cracked the glass. Angry at his cracked windshield, he reached over me, opened my door, and pushed me out of the truck and into the street. Rocks and pebbles pelted me all over as Bruce spun off without me. My mind was racing. What had I done to make him so angry? It frightened me to see that handsome face contorted into an evil rage. I tried to stand. My head hurt and was bleeding. When I looked down the open road, I saw Bruce's truck coming right for me.

"My God, he's going to run me over!" I said out loud.

I silently begged God to spare my life. The truck came to a screeching halt beside me. Bruce got out of the truck and hugged me. He had tears in his eyes and told me he was sorry, and that it would never happen again. He never did tell me what he was upset about in the first place.

I was walking on eggshells in the days that followed. All my phone calls were monitored, and I wasn't allowed to be with my friends and family unless Bruce was present. I was not allowed to leave the house without him. The constant fear and trying to cover up cuts and bruises was exhausting and taking its toll on me, both mentally and physically. I broke Bruce's rules and had a friend pick up the kids and me. I had had enough. I was leaving.

Just a few short hours later, Bruce appeared. He was crying, very apologetic, and begged to speak to me. He looked so sad that I agreed to go into the hallway and talk to him. As soon as I shut the door behind me, he pummeled me with his fists until I fell to the floor, and then he proceeded to kick me while I was down. My breath gave way, and I nearly lost consciousness. He yanked me up by my arm and demanded that I get the kids and that I had five minutes to do it or else my whole family would be in body bags. I believed him. We went back.

The broken ribs nearly punctured my lung. I couldn't even hold my baby. The pain was excruciating. My fairy-tale romance had turned into a nightmare. I still got kicked, slapped, and punched every night, because the house wasn't clean enough and the meals weren't good enough. The added violence was hindering my healing process. I was going through the motions like a robot. Misery and despair permeated my being.

We moved into a first-floor apartment in the city. Then Bruce lost his business somewhere along the line. I was too afraid to ask how. I had suspected he was using drugs for quite some time, but I wasn't sure. Money was tight. There was no heat, hot water, or telephone. I was relieved that Bruce didn't hang around the house much. Sometimes, he wouldn't come home for a couple of days at a time. I hoped and prayed he would never come back, but he always did. It was not knowing when that would cause me the greatest anxiety. I was afraid of what he might do to me and the kids if I left again. I knew he could kill us.

I always feared Bruce, but I didn't realize that I was in danger from other men as well. One night, I had closed the heavy sliding wooden doors, which led to the living room, and locked the back door. Suddenly, we were awakened by someone loudly banging on the back door. When Bruce got up to answer the door, three men barged in. One man held onto me while the other two men began violently beating Bruce with clubs, right in front of my eyes. The streetlight cast a soft beam of light between the windowsill and the shade. I was unhurt, but I watched in horror as Bruce was severely beaten. I wondered if he would die. Even though I sometimes hated this man, I did not want to see him killed. The men left quickly, and the sounds of car doors slamming and tires screeching filled the night. Bruce and I didn't talk the rest of the night. I was afraid to speak to him.

The next day, I worked up the courage to ask Bruce if he knew why the events of the previous evening had happened. He told me that the men thought he had stolen some drugs from them but swore they got the wrong man. Bruce handed me some money and told me to go out and buy a gun. Owing to some misunderstanding, he wasn't allowed to purchase a gun under his own name. I did not want a gun around with small children in the house, but Bruce promised that the gun would stay under the sink and the clip would be on top of the refrigerator. I relented and bought the gun. I hoped and prayed that things would be okay.

Two weeks later, Bruce came home drunk and in a very bad mood. He demanded that I have a beer with him while I listened to his tirades about how "you and your brats are making me broke...." Bruce began to beat me, throwing me all over the house and overturning furniture. He slammed me so hard into the wall that it left an imprint. Blinding pain wracked my body with each blow. I ran to the door to try to escape his rage. As soon as I touched the doorknob, I felt the ice-cold barrel of the gun pressed tightly against my temple.

I was terrified and sobbing uncontrollably. My life flashed before my eyes. I prayed for strength, and once again, I prayed for my life. I had to think fast. I wanted to live. I wanted my children to live. I forced myself to look into his eyes, which were now darting back and forth like those of a crazed, trapped animal, and started talking to him, telling him everything he wanted to hear. I told him how sorry I was and that everything was my fault. I promised that I would never make him angry again if he would please put down the gun. When he lowered the gun to the floor, I ran across the kitchen and literally dove through the screen and out the open window. I had no choice but to leave the kids in the house, but he had never harmed them in the past, only me, so I prayed they would be safe. I ran as fast as I could to the nearest pay phone and called the police. Then I walked slowly back to the house, and by the time I got to the driveway, the police were arriving.

I saw three police officers walk up my driveway. I walked into the house with them. There were two males and one female. I tried to explain what had happened the best that I could. When we walked into the house, I couldn't believe my eyes. Bruce had cleaned up the whole apartment. He was cool, calm, and collected. One of the male officers said, "There don't seem to be any signs of a struggle."

The male officers eyed me suspiciously.

Bruce piped up and said, "Smell her breath. She's crazy and drunk. I have to deal with this all the time. She even put a gun to my head!"

After hearing that, I was on the verge of hysterics, while Bruce sat calmly with a smile on his face. One of the male officers informed me that he was going to keep my gun and lectured me about my drinking problem and how I could've killed somebody, while the other two officers were searching the apartment with flashlights.

"Look at this," the female officer said, while shining the flashlight on my body imprint on the wall. "She's telling the truth." Hope returned to my soul for the first time in months. Someone believed me!

The police made Bruce leave the house for twenty-four hours. It was the first time ever that he was made to leave, even though he stayed in his car on the side of the road, with the engine running all night, to make sure I didn't leave. I was glad anyway. It was still twenty-four hours without him in my sight.

I've thought about that female police officer every day since then. She saved my life. She opened my eyes to see my situation for what it was: to kill or to be killed. Either way, there would be no winners.

A month later, one evening Bruce was bored. There was no money for bars and drugs. I was grateful that he was in a mellow mood. Bruce told me to go to the library and get him something to read and not to take too long, or else. A thought occurred to me.

"This may be my last chance. I've got to act now, and fast!"

I ran to the library and grabbed a few books without even glancing at the titles. I checked the books out and ran across town to a property management business that rents apartments. I very quickly explained my situation, and they agreed to help me as soon as I applied for welfare. I couldn't believe my good fortune. There would be no stopping me now. I ran back home with the books, with Bruce none the wiser.

I put all my fear aside and asked the lady across the street for help. She is an older parent with a special needs child whose son had often played with my kids in the yard. She allowed me the use of her phone over a two-week period and watched my kids while I went out to apply for welfare, got to the courthouse to get a protection-from-abuse order, and secured the apartment, with key in hand.

On the day I finally had everything arranged, believe it or not, my former husband and his parents were the ones to secretly move our furniture and things to our new place. We rushed so fast, not knowing when Bruce would return, we broke a number of items, but at that point, I didn't care. I only took what furniture was absolutely needed, such as the kids' beds, a television, a couch, dressers, and a kitchen table. They brought over a few boxes that they had, and we were throwing everything into trash bags.

The kids and I rode over in Robert's mother's car, and Robert and his dad brought the truck with our belongings. We hurriedly unloaded the truck, and the people in our building, men, women, and even some of the kids began helping us unload and carry things up the stairs. While thanking them all for their help, I related what had happened and why we were there.

The neighbors living directly below me told me to jump up and down as hard as I could and they would immediately call the police. My new neighbors assured me again and again not to worry. They told me they would get him before he got me. I felt so reassured by their support, that it gave me the courage to complete the move. They might never really know how instrumental they were in giving me the final boost I needed to put aside my fear and do what I needed to do to save my life and to protect my kids.

My hands shook with anticipation as I struggled to put the key in the lock of my new third-floor apartment, with my children and our meager belongings in tow. The door opened to one of the most beautiful sights I had ever seen. A wonderful warped floor with torn linoleum and a leaky faucet.

It was much more than that. It represented freedom from fear and violence and an opportunity for a second chance at life. No matter where I live, and whatever abundance I am lucky enough to come into, I will always remember that rundown apartment, which through another's eyes might have been seen as pitiful but was a castle in mine. It was not just a place to live. It was a whole new start on my life, for me and my children.

This story began in the summer of 1988 and ended in 1990. Bruce found Penny in a short time—she never found out how—and made only one attempt to get into her home. As they had promised her, the men in her building thwarted Bruce's attempts. He never bothered Penny or the children again. Penny is now happily married to her husband, Richard, who patiently endured the arduous process it took Penny to trust and love another man. Penny still maintains friendships with the neighbors who protected her. Richard is the brother of one of those neighbors. They were friends first, but then developed a special bond. They are now enjoying each other, and life with their six children.

Eleven-Plus

Rayelenn Sparks Casey

*T*he boy was only eleven. Squinty-eyed, knobby-kneed, topped with a tousled mass of tangled blond curls, he still wore the short trousers and tall socks that marked a boy as still a child in Yorkshire, England, in the mid-1950s. He looked forward eagerly to the day he would "drop," the day he'd first wear long trousers and be considered a grown-up. He didn't look forward, however, to the eleven-plus exam.

The idea of giving an examination to eleven-year-old children that would unalterably define their future lives is unbelievable to most Americans. But for generations, children in England viewed the eleven-plus exam as the great divider. Its purpose was to separate those who showed potential for university and future professional work from those who did not. Its very existence was based on a theory, determined by research sponsored by the British government, that by age eleven, one's IQ was set for life.

Designed as a selection test to sift out those who would go on to the highly academic "grammar" schools from those who would not, it was touted as a fair way to ensure that children were selected for the academic schools on the basis of merit, not family wealth or influence. However, the very fact that children of the rich and influential had access to better educational opportunities before age eleven meant the test was routinely passed mostly by children of privilege.

Year after year, for decades, children sat the eleven-plus exam; fewer than 25 percent of those children actually received passes and went on to grammar school. The rest, barred at age eleven from any hopes for university education, were thereby also barred from professional careers.

The boy was a good child, a quiet child. He had dreaded every day of school for as long as he could remember, but he worked hard and did his best. Outside of school, he was a voracious reader. He was an aircraft enthusiast; he could identify every kind of aircraft by its silhouette or even the sound of its engines, and he knew a lot about how they worked, too. But in school, no one would have called him academically gifted. He did his sums, completed his spelling and grammar assignments, learned the capitals and major exports of the countries of the world. He got middling grades, and usually ranked somewhere near the bottom of the class. He feared the masters too much to engage them in the kind of conversation that might have let them guess at his true potential, but he got by.

He didn't pin any real hopes on the exam. Lads at the bottom of the class just didn't. Frankly, most of the children at his school approached the day assuming they'd not pass. There were stories of children from his kind of background surprising everyone by passing the eleven-plus and winning educational opportunities. But most held no such hope.

That year, the year he was eleven, school dragged on in its normal way. Playing cricket and making model airplanes were his passions; school was the burden that, being a child, he must endure. The time for the exam loomed near, and, if he thought about it at all, it was with a mixture of hopelessness and resignation.

The day came for the head of school to announce the date and time of the test and to distribute the permission slips that each child's parents had to sign. A hush came over the boy's class when the headmaster entered the room. As he strode through the door, the boy and his classmates stood as one, as they had been taught; they sat obediently when he told them to sit. He was a kindly man, recognized as both strict and fair, widely known to be one of the best headmasters in the city. But they knew his authority, and so they did not fiddle with the pen nibs and pots of ink, did not shuffle their feet, did not whisper or giggle. The boy's teacher moved to one side, yielding to the head, who briskly marched to the front of the room and stood against the chalkboard, hands grasped behind his back in the age-old stance of headmasters.

The headmaster announced the upcoming test and described its three parts: sums, reading skills, and reasoning. He outlined how the test would be administered, and when. And then the headmaster gently told the boy's class that, in his opinion, it was unlikely that anyone in the class would pass the test. In fact, he suggested quietly, it was a bit of a waste of time for any of them to sit the exam. But he handed out the permission slips and instructed the children to tell their parents everything he had said. If anyone's parents still wished for them to take the test, they were welcome to return the permission slip the next day.

The boy went home and told his mum exactly what the headmaster had said—that, in his opinion, it was unlikely that any of the children would pass the test, that it seemed a waste of time for them to take it, but that they could sit the exam if their parents wanted them to.

His mother considered his words judiciously. In her time and place and understanding, the headmaster, like the doctor and the solicitor, was a man of wisdom and authority. One respected the headmaster, and so one respected his opinion. If he believed that none of the children in her boy's class would pass the exam, she reasoned, it must be true. After all, he was the headmaster. Why waste her son's time or the school's. She did not sign the permission slip.

The boy did not take the test. None of the children in his classroom took the test. He did not go on to grammar school, where he would have been given the academic preparation for university. He stayed in his school until he was fifteen, learning enough mathematics and writing skills to be a good tradesman. His mother, through her excellent connections, found him the opportunity to sign on as an apprentice with a painter/decorator. It was a skilled trade with a good future, and the boy did very well. His boss took an interest in him, and gave him excellent training, and the boy successfully completed his seven-year apprenticeship.

For many children in England, that would have been the end of the story—a steady job for life. But during the first year of his employment as a skilled painter and decorator, this boy woke up one day and said to himself, "I do not wish to be a tradesman all my life."

Still airplane crazy, the boy dared to give up his newly acquired trade and accept an entry-level job selling airline tickets in a local airport. Eighteen months later, the boy who never took the eleven-plus exam was named a manager of that airline. The boy who never took the eleven-plus exam served as an executive in the British aviation industry for almost twenty years, running successively larger and busier and more influential stations for the United Kingdom's second largest airline, eventually training graduates of Oxford University and being asked to start a whole new business for his company.

Then, at age forty, sensing a call to ordained ministry, the boy who never took the eleven-plus exam moved to America, enrolled in Gettysburg College in Gettysburg, Pennsylvania, and graduated magna cum laude, the top-ranking student in both the philosophy and the religion departments; he was elected to Phi Beta Kappa. Three years later, he completed a master of divinity degree from Virginia Theological Seminary.

The boy who never took the eleven-plus exam is now a fifty-five-year-old Episcopal priest. He is an insightful thinker, superb writer, skilled debater, trusted counselor, and wise leader. He is respected by many as an intellect and a scholar. He is my husband, the Reverend Stephen Casey.

There is something indomitable in the spirit of each of us, something that allows us to soar above the barriers and find our true home. Finding that indomitable something deep within requires creativity and openness; acting on it requires courage and singleness of heart. Stephen, refusing to succumb to cultural and societal barriers, found his true home, and in so doing is an inspiration to the many who know him.

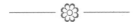

Rayelenn Sparks Casey is a teacher, writer, and professional sign-language interpreter living in Lancaster, Pennsylvania, with Stephen, her husband, and their daughters, Emily and Elizabeth. They all share a love of learning and a belief that there is always something worth striving for just ahead.

Amazing Hands

Roland Hays

My mother-in-law, Grandma Hayes, led my four-year-old nephew, Mal, through Grand Central Railway station. It was enormous, with echoes bouncing like Ping-Pong balls, from one wall to another. Mal was in awe of everything he heard. The train announcer's voice reverberated into the corners and crevices of the domed ceiling and back. Every two or three minutes a rumble lifted from beneath the floor, and Mal could feel the tremble as another train arrived and departed. Shrill whistles denoted the conductors' signaling engineers. Passengers shuffled about, lifting, dropping, and pulling luggage, rushing to get to their trains on time. Rustle, slap, slide. Rustle, slap, slide.

There were odors too that delighted Mal's nose. A familiar aroma wafted over from the popcorn stall. Slightly sickening smells of coffee and sweet rolls mingled with those of the spicy mustard and pickles from the snack bar. A pungent grease scent hovered over the hamburger grill.

Mal was transfixed by all there was to see. Vendors hawked springy, feathery Kewpie dolls and bouncy balloons on sticks. A wrinkled, hunchbacked newsstand attendant struggled to undo a bundle of magazines that kept sliding from his grasp. A man and woman in a corner made strange gestures at each other. A group of teenagers danced across the room to a jazz beat from a booming radio one of them carried on his shoulder. Their heads bobbed, and their hands slapped their thighs as they gyrated back and forth, two steps forward, three steps backward. Mal wondered if they'd ever get to where they were going.

Then Mal's eyes fell on something he'd never seen before. He froze in his spot, staring, trying to assimilate what he saw. It looked like a man riding a broad scooter, but not a whole man. A half man. A man with no legs.

The man was maneuvering his upper body on the scooter with his hands. He smiled and nodded at passersby as he sped along at a lively clip. The man was a skillful driver. Not once did he bump anyone or run into anything, quite unlike Mal, who often collided with things when he rode his bike around the playground. The man's body was broad and muscular. His neck was thick and his arms were large and hairy. In each gloved hand he held a wooden block, a rubber cushion attached to the bottom. With these pressed against the floor, he scooted along with an air of gaiety.

Mal was fascinated. He slipped his hand from his grandmother's (no easy feat, but accomplished because she was preoccupied with looking for the right subway exit) and ran over to the man.

"Hi. Whatcha doin'?" Mal asked.

"Why, I'm going to work," the man answered jovially.

"You are? What kinda work do you do?"

The man laughed. "I'm a salesman. I sell pencils." He pointed to a can set in a holder on the front of his scooter. The can was full of pencils—colorful, new, and orderly. Beside the can was a change maker attached to the scooter frame by a sturdy chain to insure safety from vandals.

"Wow!" exclaimed Mal appreciatively, his eyes and face beaming, showing the respect he felt. "Your hands can walk and work too!"

Rebecca lives in Scottsdale, Arizona. Although a retired teacher, she continues to work with children as a substitute in the school system, in the children's ministry at her church, and with Native American children on the reservation. She writes children's picture-book stories along with her memoirs and adult essays. Four children and five grandchildren continually feed her ideas for her stories.

Mal, like the "half-man," overcame many difficulties in his life, and now designs African American jewelry and artwork. Mal's appreciation for beauty and for his African American culture enabled him to overcome his obstacles.

My Cup Runneth Over

Roberta Victor

*I*was twenty-seven years young. George and I had been married a mere six months. And for a few weeks, he had been angry all the time, provoking an argument at every opportunity. It was late at night, and we were caught driving in the pouring rain. George was trying to argue. I was trying to ignore him. We came up on a sharp curve in the road. Just before the curve, George shouted and then lunged at me. He had never hurt me, so I was completely unprepared for what followed. He snapped my neck with both of his hands. One hand held my neck firmly, while the other hand snapped my head in a quick pushing motion, which caused lateral sheering of my spinal column.

I could feel and hear the bones cracking. George was trained in hand-to-hand combat during his military service in Vietnam. The neck snap is usually fatal. When he let go of the steering wheel to assault me, the car flipped twice and landed upside down in a ditch.

I remember being amazed that I could see my back where my chest should have been and registering what that meant. My neck was broken. My head was turned completely around. My chin was resting in the hood of my car coat. I have seen the newspaper clipping with the photograph showing this, and my physician later confirmed that it was a miracle that I survived such a devastating injury.

I could not move. Not just because of the way I was pinned in the car, but because I was paralyzed from the neck down.

I heard the ambulance arrive. I heard the emergency crew talking to me. It seemed to take forever for them to get me out of the car, put me on the stretcher, and get me into the ambulance. From the emergency room, I was admitted to the intensive care unit. When the neurosurgeon confirmed that I was paralyzed from the neck down, I was devastated. When he told me that George was on his way home to see about my son, my paralysis took a back seat to my concern for my son's safety. My precious six-year-old son, Shannon, could be in harm's way from the man who had just broken my neck.

I could do nothing about it but hope that someone would protect him. My life as I knew it was changed forever. I gave the doctor my neighbor's and my parents' phone number. After what seemed like an eternity, the doctor reassured me that he had spoken to my neighbor and my parents and that my son would be kept safe.

The next thing I knew, my mother was waking me up. She assured me that my son was safe and sound in the waiting room with my father. My parents would take Shannon home to stay with them until I could come home from the hospital. I asked to see my son. The nurse said he was too young to come into the intensive care unit. I knew I could not let myself sink into despair, for my son's sake. I visited with my mother and told her to give Shannon a big hug from me. She left and as I drifted off to sleep again, I did what I have always done: I counted my blessings. I was alive. I was able to think, talk, see, and hear. There was hope that surgery would restore me to full mobility.

As I thought about all these things, I saw a vision of myself with a beautiful cup raised high over my head. I tipped the cup just a fraction, and crystal clear water poured down my arms into my face. "My cup runneth over." I murmured these words over and over again: "My cup runneth over."

I had no intention of accepting this paralysis. I did not have time for this! Twenty days later, the neurosurgeon told me the X-rays were finally clear. Two cervical vertebrae were crushed. My spinal chord looked like a Zorro sign and was crimped but not severed. He described the surgical procedure he believed would restore my mobility. He would take the pointed part of my pelvic bone and fashion two vertebrae to replace the crushed ones.

The surgery restored mobility to my upper body, but from the waist down, I was still paralyzed. I was very mindful of the blessing of even half-body mobility, but I was not willing to settle for that. My cup was half full ... but the vision I had was of a cup running over.

The beautiful vision I had kept getting clouded by other thoughts running obsessively through my mind. I broke into a sweat when I saw myself, over and over again, in the car and felt George snapping my neck. The awful reality that I might not ever play with my son again, walk again, or dance again, began to sink in. Then, I remembered the vision of me tipping the cup running over with water. I disciplined my mind to see myself playing with my son, walking, working, doing all kinds of everyday things, and dancing. Every time I would begin to worry or feel a dark cloud of hopelessness, I would make myself think about all of the things that I would never take for granted again, and that which I looked forward to doing again.

I began the long journey of physical therapy. I thought that before I could dance, I would start small, with the goal of walking to the bathroom. I was tired of bedpans. I asked the nurse to scoot me down to the foot of the bed, so that my feet touched the metal of the bed frame. I figured that if I could concentrate on feeling the metal against my feet, the muscles and nerves in my body would have to wake up. She shrugged, frowned, and called in another nurse to help. After they moved me, I sat up so I could see that my feet were touching the foot of the bed.

I focused on feeling the metal. I felt my energy pouring into the nerves on the bottoms of my feet. Every waking moment, the bottoms of my feet became my only focal point. Four days later, I woke up in the middle of the night.

My feet felt like they were on fire! Still half asleep, I cried out in pain. Then I realized what this meant. My feet were burning with the sensation of nerves waking up after a long sleep. I shouted into the nurses' intercom, "I can feel my feet!"

Within seconds, I heard the thunder of footsteps in the hall. Two nurses came in my room. I showed them that I could wiggle my toes just the tiniest bit. I could feel my legs waking up. I said, "I have to go to the bathroom. Help me walk."

I was determined to walk to the bathroom now. So the nurses helped me to the edge of the bed. They held me up as I struggled to my feet. As soon as my feet touched the floor, I expected to stand up easily. My legs folded under me as if I were a rag doll. I told the nurses to just help me down to the floor. I would crawl before I would use a bedpan again.

I crawled to the bathroom and pulled myself up onto the commode. I was so thrilled with this accomplishment. I was barefoot. The floor felt deliciously cold to my feet. It was as if the very nerve endings and skin on the bottom of my feet were celebrating. I crawled back to my bed. I was triumphant and very tired.

Before I drifted back to sleep, I thanked God for helping me stay strong in my mind and spirit, even though my body was weak and broken. In the morning, I began to do everything I could to strengthen my legs. The doctor came into my room. This was a triumphant moment. He began to outline the treatment and exercises I needed to do in order to be discharged. As soon as I could walk the hall up and back twice with no help, I could go home.

The process of learning to walk again and strengthen my upper body while the muscles healed unfolded slowly and painstakingly over the next several days. Finally, early one morning, I made it! As I finished the home stretch and approached the nursing station, a few other nurses came out into the hall and began to applaud.

Just then, my doctor walked out of the elevator across from the nursing station. He could tell by the expression on my face that I had just "made the grade" to go home. He reached into his pocket, pulled out a small tape recorder, placed it on the counter of the nursing station, and turned it on.

"Moon River" began to play. He bowed and held his hand out to me saying, "I believe this is our dance."

There I stood ... in an ungainly, awkward breastplate back brace ... with tufts of what very little hair I had (bright orange from frequent Betadine washes every day) sticking out in a way that would make Emmett Kelly green with envy. My scalp was shaved where they stitched the cuts from the windshield glass of the car and the stitches from my surgery. My face was still bruised, and makeup was of little help. I was wearing a long, frumpy robe, but ... I felt like the belle of the ball.

I stepped forward, and my doctor and I danced. I felt awkward at first. Within a few steps, I felt light as a feather and in my glory. Hope took wings and lifted me into the sweet, lazy rhythm of "Moon River." Tears of joy streamed down my face as I danced the dance of triumph over tragedy. I would dance. Oh, yes. I would dance right out of this hospital in just a few days.

I spent the next three days in physical therapy, learning how to navigate life in this ponderous neck brace. After thirty-six days in the hospital, the day finally came ... I was going home.

I was staying with my parents for the time it would take to heal and strengthen from the surgery and the trauma of what had happened to me. That was a real challenge. My father became even more emotionally and verbally controlling and abusive than he was when I was a child. Just days before the divorce was final, George called me and told me he was attending Alcoholics Anonymous meetings and church. He begged my forgiveness and for a chance to prove he had changed.

My discernment was very distorted by the constant brutal truculence I was now enduring every day from my father. Only those who have known and endured the emotional wearing down from constant verbal abuse can truly grasp how reconciling with George made sense to me at the time. I agreed to give our love and life together another chance. We found an apartment and had a decent and hopeful life for about two years. During that time, I gave birth to my beloved daughter, Amanda, the most precious blessing to come from the attempt at reconciliation with George. I carried her through full term with no complications, a true miracle from God.

When Amanda was five weeks old, George started drinking again and became violent. I immediately filed criminal charges against George (he was put on three years of probation and released), filed for divorce, and began my life anew with my son, Shannon, age nine, and daughter, Amanda, a newborn.

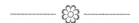

Twenty-two years later, Roberta is now fifty-two years young and shares her life with the composer Robin Blankenship. She is a writer and storyteller. She and Robin work together producing CDs of Robin's music and of her storytelling and inspirational narrations, accompanied by Robin's music.

The $4,000,000 Question

Robin L. Silverman

*I*n 1997, a major flood devastated our town of Grand Forks, North Dakota, destroying homes, businesses, houses of worship, schools, and more in its wake. The victims turned to our newly formed interfaith coalition for help with rebuilding their homes and their lives.

We were a well-intentioned group of volunteer clergy and laypeople from thirty-two evangelical, Protestant, and Catholic churches and the city's only synagogue. Our role in the city's recovery was shaped by the other federal and local service agencies, which suggested that we become the "end of the line" for people who had already been evaluated for need but had exhausted all the help the traditional social service system could offer. We eagerly accepted our role, but we had one rather large problem: we didn't have a single penny in our treasury.

We would start every meeting in prayer: "God, give us wisdom, strength, and understanding." These were wonderful qualities, but we couldn't use them for currency in the lumberyard. While we prayed, the file folders piled up. We had no money even for essentials like the light and phone bill for the tiny office space the coalition had rented.

After several weeks, I walked into the executive director's office and saw the pile of folders groaning from its own weight. I asked, "How much money will it take to help these people?"

He sighed wearily. "I don't know. Maybe $100,000."

At that point, he might as well have said one million dollars. Without financial resources, it was all the same. Then I looked up and noticed a sign tacked on the bulletin board by his desk. It read, "Trust me, Terry. I have everything under control." It was signed, "God."

I thought about the sign for a minute, and then turned to the assembled executive committee, a group composed of half a dozen clergy and a few laypeople, including me. "I think we should ask God for $100,000," I said.

There was a chorus of "Oh, no!" and "We couldn't possibly do that!" Sensing that their resistance lay in the ancient concern that money is the root of all evil, I simply asked, "Why not? Wisdom, strength, and understanding aren't helping these people. They need their houses rebuilt, and we can't do that without lumber, Sheetrock, and stuff we have to buy in a hardware store."

From deep inside the group, I heard one of the clergy say, "You know, the money isn't for us." Another echoed, "It's to help those who hurt."

"That's right," I chimed in. "It's not like we're going to take a trip to Bermuda on it. We all know it will be used for the right reasons and people."

The clergy huddled and talked it over while I watched and waited hopefully. "Okay," said one as he broke from the group. "Let's ask."

A little timidly, he began, "Lord, in your wisdom, we ask that you bring us $100,000 to buy the materials necessary to rebuild the homes of the people you have delivered to us. We promise to be your faithful servants in this task, using the money only for their good."

A few other people spoke words of promise and faith, and together we all said, "Amen."

One week later, our cup was overflowing. We had $100,000. It came to us from all kinds of people and places, but there it was, every glorious penny we had requested. In the meantime, volunteers from around the country were arriving to do the physical labor of reconstructing the houses. Work began in earnest.

Still, the requests kept coming. We had underestimated. The $100,000 barely scratched the surface of what was needed. Although the city received disaster aid, very little of it went to individuals. Worse, many hundreds of families in the rural areas lost necessities like wells and septic systems, which were poisoned or crushed by the toxic water. Replacing basics like these cost tens of thousands of dollars, and the farm economy had been bad. Without the help of our coalition, many people would be forced to exist only with bottled water and outhouses—or worse.

Realizing this, one of the evangelical pastors said, "Who are we to play small, when God obviously wants us to play big?" And with that, he started to pray, "Lord, we are your willing servants. Use us. Bring to us *all* the people who need our help, and *all* the resources, financial and otherwise, to do the work that's ours to do."

Again, together we said, "Amen!"

We should have known what would happen next, but nothing could have prepared us for the $2,000,000 check we received from an anonymous donor two months later. Better still, Lutheran Brotherhood said they would match any donations we received. They were probably thinking of a number around $50,000, but to their credit, they matched the entire $2,000,000. Our destitute coalition went from a budget of zero to one of well over $4,000,000!

And that's not all. The city donated hotel rooms for the volunteer workers. We logged more than a million nights over the next three years as good people from around the country came on their own time and dime to dig trenches, reconstruct buildings, and recement lives that had fallen apart. Ninety-eight percent of the money received went directly to buy lumber and other materials. The remaining 2 percent paid the office bills and a small stipend for the executive director, who had given up his regular job to oversee the coalition's work.

From the experience, I learned that human beings are filled to overflowing with love, hope, and promise. When we cannot see that, it is simply because we are looking in the wrong direction. When we reconnect what is right within ourselves with the loving power that created us all, all that we need—and everything we didn't even know we needed—floods into our lives.

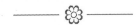

Robin L. Silverman is the author of *The Ten Gifts* and *Something Wonderful Is About to Happen.* She lives in North Dakota with her husband and two daughters.

Quest for Fame

Robin Ryan

*L*ife holds so many ironies, twists, and turns. You often wonder, where did this start and how did I get here?

For me, I think it all started with being the eighteen-month-older sister to identical twin boys. They were so cute, so adorable, and so noticed by everybody. I'm sure a psychologist could have a field day pondering the effects of being a child showered with the mommy-is-all-mine attention and then having it all abruptly end.

As fate would have it, I grew up in a large extended family with sixty-three cousins and a small town of five thousand people who were all enamored of the twins! They were impossible to tell apart. Even my father mixed them up sometimes. Everybody stopped and noticed the twins. *Everybody!*

Being part of this family influenced me to want to be noticed in a big way. Life, I have learned, is made up of choices. I had made mine early on. I would be famous, recognized, known. I took up cheerleading, being club president, lots of out-there activities, all in the quest to stand out.

This overwhelming drive for recognition propelled me as I began to develop my career. I kept trying to achieve more and more recognition in my career as an author, career counselor, and professional speaker. The more I accomplished, the more recognition I craved. Sometimes, wanting to be noticed brought out dislike from others, instead of the adoration I wanted. Yet I was so focused on fame, that for me being noticed and known was the be-all and end-all.

I wrote books, was on television and radio, and even appeared as a guest on Oprah. My name was in magazines, my books were in bookstores, the hometown paper wrote about me often, eclipsed by two major front-page feature articles written on me in the big city paper where I currently live. Recognition was short-lived acknowledgment, which simply inspired me to try harder and do more.

I was so obsessed with building my career that I put off having children, convinced that a baby would trap me and not give me the time I wanted to drive my career forward and achieve the big-time fame that was always around the corner. I kept at it, and at forty-two, I had three new books published, though only a few friends and family very briefly acknowledged it.

Be careful what you wish for, for indeed you may get it. Finally, at the age of forty-two, I got the calls, cards, letters, presents, and the avalanche of attention I had been seeking. The irony is, it wasn't from being on a television show or from gracing the cover of a magazine, nor was it a major newspaper write-up. No, it was the simple fact that at forty-two years old and after eighteen years of marriage I was having a baby.

It happens to women every day. Yet it was people's reactions that astounded me. Some were thrilled, downright ecstatic. When I told our neighbor ladies at a small function, one woman had to grab the table for support falling down from the shock. Friends screamed, simply overjoyed with the news. Even guys with whom I went to college who had never written me in twenty years since graduation, sent cards, gifts, and toys. People I didn't even know wrote and sent baby things when others who knew me told them I was having our first baby after eighteen years of marriage. I was swamped with attention. With so much emphasis on my career, everyone we knew had given up on us ever having any children.

Nothing prepared me for the celebrity status I achieved when our son was born. The excitement and adoration from so many, along with more than one hundred gifts and multitudes of cards and letters, was more than I ever could have imagined.

I was enamored all right, but here's a confession: it wasn't the attention that I had been craving that won my heart. I was completely and thoroughly mesmerized with this tiny little bundle I held in my arms. I was holding a miracle, God's greatest blessing.

After forty years of searching to get my deepest inner emotional needs satisfied, and thinking fame would do it, I came face-to-face with the reality that no outside recognition would ever complete me like having a child does. Giving birth to my son gave me my true meaning in life, and it wasn't televised.

Now when someone asks, "What do you do?" I'm not as apt to give them my résumé or brag about my best-selling books. I might just pull out the latest baby picture. My son, Jack Michael Ryan, is without question the most important accomplishment of my life.

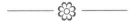

Robin Ryan is a career counselor, national speaker, and author of four best-sellers. She is grateful every day to be blessed with a wonderful son, Jack Michael Ryan, and this story is dedicated to him.

"I'm a Good Girl"

Roger Kiser

One evening after work I stopped at a local restaurant in British Columbia and ordered a hamburger, french fries, and a cup of coffee. Several minutes later a young girl, about eighteen or nineteen years old, came into the restaurant and sat down beside me. She said not a word but just sat there staring at me the entire time I was trying to eat. I could see through the corner of my eye that she was looking at me, so I acted as though I did not notice her.

"Are you going to eat all those fries?" she finally asked me.

I looked up at her face and saw that she was rather thin and quite an attractive young lady.

"Are you hungry?" I asked.

"I haven't eaten nothing since yesterday morning," she responded.

I noticed that several of her teeth were missing. The ones that she had left were not far from meeting a dentist's pliers. I motioned to the cook and I asked him to please prepare the young lady a hamburger, fries, and a Coke. I was quite shocked when she told me that she could pay me for the meal.

"Why would you want my leftover fries if you could buy your own?" I asked her.

"I always pay my own way," she said, as she reached over and unbuttoned the top button of her blouse and then looked down at the floor.

"Are you a prostitute?" I asked her.

"Not really," she replied. "But a man's gotta do what a man's gotta do," she mumbled.

I turned and looked directly at her face and she said, "That's just an expression that we girls use out on the streets."

I told her that I was married and that no payment was necessary. I also told her that I would be willing to meet with her, now and then, as I was planning to write a story about life on the street and that I would be willing to pay her a little something for her time, as well as her story.

"Could I have $25 now?" she asked.

I looked at her, thought for a moment, and then handed her the money.

"When can we meet again?" I asked her.

"Same time tomorrow?" she replied.

"Okay. I will see you then," I said, as I got up and left the restaurant.

I stood around the corner until she came out of the restaurant and then I followed her until I saw her enter the front door of a small fleabag located in the worst part of town.

When I returned to the restaurant the next day, there was no sign of the young lady. I waited two hours for her to appear, then headed for her hotel. I described her to the clerk, who wouldn't disclose any information about their "upstanding guest" until I put $10 on the counter.

"She is my sister, and I need to find her *now*!" I yelled at him.

"Room 211," he said, pointing toward the stairway.

Slowly I walked up the stairs and found the room. I knocked on the door, but no one answered. I knocked again and the door slowly opened, just a crack.

"What do you want?" said the girl, as she turned her face from me.

I pushed the door open and entered the room.

"Thought we had a meeting," I said. "I would like my money back."

She ran over to the small, unmade bed, fell across it, and began to sob. Not knowing what to do, I walked over and sat down on the edge of the bed. I slowly lowered my hand onto her back and began to rub, softly, back and forth. When she finally turned over onto her back I could see that her mouth was somewhat bloody and that she had two black eyes.

"Who did this?" I asked her.

"John," she replied.

"Who is John?"

"The man who runs this hotel, the guy downstairs."

I learned that she had come to Vancouver from Moose Jaw, Saskatchewan, several months before, and that she had met John in the same restaurant where we had met. She was broke, and John had told her that he would give her a free room and that he could show her how to make "lots of money." When she had told him "I'm a good girl," and had refused to become a prostitute, he devised a scheme to get money from men by having her sit in the restaurant, hour after hour, until men would approach her. She would have them pay her for sex but she would just sit there until the men got frustrated and would leave without sex or their money. John beat her up when she didn't come back to the hotel with enough money to make him happy.

"I just want to go back home," she kept crying. I got up from the bed, and I told her to pack her few belongings. I walked over to the small dresser and opened the drawers, one after the other, but they were totally bare. "Go down to the bathroom and clean up. I'll be back in a minute," I told her.

When I reached the bottom of the stairs, I looked directly at the man sitting behind the counter.

"Are you John?" I asked.

"Yes," he replied.

"Do you believe in prayer?" I asked.

"Not really," he told me.

"That's a real shame, my friend," I stated, as I walked toward him. He jumped up from behind the counter and ran into a small room and locked the door. I looked up and saw the girl walking down the stairs. I began to knock on the door, and I told John that he and I had a date and that I would wait for as long as it took for him to come out.

I walked over to the counter and noticed that the cash register was open. I took out $25 and I stuck the money in my front pocket. As I sat down in John's chair my foot hit something beneath the desk. When I looked I noticed a small cash box. I picked up the box and sat it on top of the desk. I opened the metal box and found pictures of six girls and cash totaling about $14,000.

"Do you know any of these girls?" I asked my new friend.

"They're out working the streets," she replied.

"Can you find them, real fast?" I asked her.

"I think so."

For the next hour I continually knocked on the door trying to get John to come out, but he refused. Within the hour, four of the six girls returned and were sitting on the floor, waiting to see what I was going to do. After an hour, I figured I'd given John a long enough chance to show his face.

I got up from the chair and walked outside, where I saw a man drinking from a bottle wrapped in a brown paper bag. I told him that I would give him $100 if he would sit in the chair and knock on the door every five minutes without saying a word, which he agreed to do.

I took the girls, along with the $14,000, down to a local department store, where I purchased them each a new suitcase, toothbrush, makeup, purse, and new clothing. I also purchased each of them a bus ticket to anywhere that they wanted to go. Inside each of the purses I placed $2,000 in cash.

I shook hands with the girls as they all boarded the bus together, heading to Kamloops, to get them out of Vancouver and away from John.

The last girl to enter the bus was the one I had met at the restaurant several days before. She looked at me, and I winked at her. We said not a word as she walked up the steps and sat down in the front of the bus. As the bus pulled out of the station I saw her look back at me and wave. I raised my thumb into the air, nodded my head forward, and I silently motioned with my lips, "Good girl."

I walked back to my car and headed home. On the way I stopped at the local supermarket, where I purchased two large lobsters, two large baking potatoes, and some broccoli for my wife and me. The $128 and odd change that remained from the $14,000 I threw out of the car window and watched it blow away in the wind.

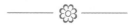

Roger Kiser is the author of the book *Orphan: A True Story of Abandonment, Abuse, and Redemption.* Roger writes short stories for *Chicken Soup for the Soul, Heartwarmers,* the *Heartwarmers of Love* book series, and the *Petwarmers* CD collection. Roger now spends most of his time writing about child abuse. He and his wife, Judy, operate the Sad Orphan Foundation. He will never forget how he and three hundred other children were treated as though they were less than human while living in a Jacksonville, Florida, orphanage.

It Will Be Good

Roiza Weinreich

I am an adult woman who has endured my share of suffering in life, just as most of us have. Throughout the natural ups and downs that occurred in my life as a child, then as a mother and wife, my parents have always been a solid source of strength and inspiration for me. When I was a young girl with a scraped knee, I remember my father encouraging me with these words: "It hurts, but it will get better quickly—it will be good. By the time you are a bride, you'll forget you ever fell." I have tripped and fallen many times in my life since becoming a bride and mother, and still, my father's words heal me.

If I could plan and prepare before disappointments, I'm sure I'd take them in stride. The problem is that they tend to come unexpected and unannounced. That's why I'm still calling my father almost every day, although his great-grandchildren are as old as I was then, for encouragement.

Just the other day I witnessed one of a thousand examples of how my father's lifelong attitude, "It will be good," spills over into his daily life, and thank God, into mine.

My parents had just arrived in their apartment in Florida the previous night. Each winter they spend about four months down south. Although thousands of people travel by plane each day I always feel a bit nervous about them traveling, so I called to check in on them. "Everything is wonderful," my father assured me. "The apartment looks lovely," my mother agreed. "The air is so pleasant. I can walk outside in November in shirtsleeves and enjoy the sunshine," my father added. "By the way," my mother commented, "the refrigerator is broken."

I felt my heart sink. I know what it's like to struggle with refrigerators that don't work. Two summers ago I rented a cabin with a fridge that needed defrosting every two weeks. My kids thought it was funny: "We're the only ones who have snow in the summer." I would blow-dry the ice to make it melt more quickly. I don't remember laughing along.

I remembered my neighbor whose fridge was broken this past summer. She had left her milk, juice, and dairy products in ours. Running back and forth between our summer homes was a hassle. My neighbor had to buy new supplies every day. At one point she said, "If they don't fix the fridge today, I'd rather go home. This just doesn't feel like a vacation."

"How are you coping?" I asked my mother, alarmed to hear the news.

I heard my mother's calm voice on the line. "Don't worry. We went out last night and bought ice and a dish-pan and put it in the refrigerator. When I lived in Argentina in the 1950s I had an icebox for two years. It'll be just fine with an icebox for a few days until the repairman comes."

"Mom, that's the perfect answer to the problem!" I exclaimed. I'm so used to having a working refrigerator that I'd be totally distraught if it suddenly broke down. I wouldn't have thought of this idea. I just want a working fridge that stays cold and no puddles on the floor, please.

I felt so proud of my parents—they are my unsung heroes. Their quiet courage helps me smile throughout the day. I wish I had the words to communicate the depth of their character, and the miracle of my mother and father's unceasing optimistic attitude toward life. Perhaps knowing about a picture will help you understand how exceptional they are.

In the dining room of my parents' home, there hangs a still life. It's not a pretty picture. It has a gray background. There is a bare table that has two large scallions, a piece of watermelon, a dark beige half loaf of bread, and some kind of crockery filled with water. That's the entire picture. As a child, and even as an adult, I always wondered why they displayed this ugly picture in the dining room.

Recently I asked. My father told me, "I left home when I was eighteen. I never saw most of my family or anyone I grew up with in Krakow ever again. I wandered from place to place. I ran away from the Nazis to Lemberg. Shortly after that, the Russians exiled all Polish citizens to Siberia.

"In Siberia we had only the threadbare clothes we wore, yet the winters were much colder than the ones we have here. A small loaf of bread was shared by four people, and that's all we had to eat for an entire day. Later we were freed, and we went southward to Samarkand. Samarkand is in the area of Uzbekistan in Russia. Even then, however, if I had as much food as is in this picture, it was a feast."

My father continued, "I like to look at this picture. It reminds me to feel grateful that God took me from there, and brought me to here."

It was Friday, and the Sabbath was soon approaching. The repairman had not come as hoped for, yet my mother still sounded like her cheerful, unflustered self. "I'm pretty sure the ice will keep things cold," she assured me. My mother's words gave me a surge of energy. I can't start my day without a dose of her optimism.

I called again on Sunday morning. My father sounded triumphant. "The ice lasted longer than expected. It kept everything cold for thirty-six hours!"

I savor that memory, hearing my father's proud voice describing how he had responded to this challenge and found a solution. My parents enjoy every hour of every day. Their happiness isn't dependent on appliances working.

About four days later the repairman came. My father's voice sang as he announced, "It's cold now inside the refrigerator! Now, things will be a little easier. I knew all along that everything would be good in the end.

"You know something, Rosie. My mother, may she rest in peace, said a compliment about me that I think of often, 'My son always says that it will be good.'"

When I fall I want someone to notice and say, "So sorry!" My father looks at it differently. He wants to get up and move on. His gratitude and unceasing optimism got him to where he is today. Out of the ashes he kept his dreams alive. Although he came to this country as a lone survivor from his family, he didn't give up. He learned a new language and new skills, built up a family and a community, and created a successful business, with only his faith in God and his resourcefulness to rely upon.

"It will be good!" That is my father's legacy. He believes it so strongly that some of the time, I believe it, too.

Roiza Weinreich is a dedicated wife, mother, teacher, and daughter and the author of several books about self-esteem and personal growth, including *W.H.A.T. Can Relieve Stress!* She lives a short distance from her mother and father and is fortunate to have daily contact with them.

All Was Not Lost, and Even More Was Found

Ronda Graby Stump

"It was the best of times. It was the worst of times." I think that's how the famous line goes. Those words sure described my life with my husband, Jim, a decade ago.

Jim and I met in college, courted for two years, and were married in September 1990. We moved into our first apartment together, pinching and saving, hoping to build our dream house within five years. Jim and I were then, and still are, each other's best friends. We have always said "roommates for life." April 1991, while still newlyweds, would be the first big test of that commitment.

It was my first night out with the girls since I'd gotten married. I left excited to see longtime friends. I remember saying, "Jim, enjoy a quiet night at home. Put your feet up and watch some baseball." My friends and I were celebrating the upcoming nuptials of our friends with a bachelorette night on the town.

After dinner, we decided to go dance-club hopping. We started dancing and toasting the upcoming wedding day, when my sister, Lori, rushed into the club unexpectedly. At first, I thought it was just a neat coincidence. I later found out she had spent the last hour and a half frantically searching all the local clubs for me. She ran up to me and shouted, "We need to go now. Your house is on fire. I think it may be gone by the time we get back!"

The drive home seemed endless, even if it was less than fifteen minutes. My heart was racing, and I felt numb all over. As we raced home, Lori assured and reassured me she'd seen Jim and he wasn't hurt. "He's okay. He's sitting on your front lawn with Mom and JoAnn." Despite Lori's attempts at reassurance, I knew I'd only start to breathe again once I had seen him.

From that moment on, everything seemed surreal. We rushed home, only to be told we had to park blocks away. We parked, jumped out of our car, and ran for what seemed like hours. All I wanted was to get to my husband. I needed to touch his face and feel his powerful, protective arms around me. Ten years later, I can still vividly recall that run through the apartment complex, searching for Jim through the crowds of emergency people, firefighters, and onlookers. When I recently watched the families frantically searching for their loved ones at the World Trade Center, I remembered how I felt that evening. All you want is to see the face of your loved one through the smoke-filled crowd.

Then, finally, through the dark, smoke-covered sky, I saw Jim. He was sitting in the middle of the grassy area in front of our home as firefighters, medical personnel, neighbors, and others hurried this way and that way. I remember he looked so still and alone in the crowd, even though many people scurried about. He just sat there, quiet and pensive. I ran to him with all my heart and soul. I ran to the safety of his arms. Words can't describe the relief I felt seeing him that moment. We hugged, I cried, and we then sat glued to each other from that moment on.

As we talked, I learned that a neighbor's gas grill had exploded and caught the whole building complex on fire. Jim had been there from the start. As he sat watching the baseball game, there was a sudden pounding on the door and someone yelling, "Get out, your house is on fire!" He ran out, not even grabbing his shoes or socks. So he sat on the ground, barefoot, watching the fire rip through our lives. He apologized many times that night (and for months later) for not grabbing special mementos like my wedding gown or our photo albums. He cursed himself for not picking up his mother's ring or the heirloom holiday ornaments before he ran out. Together, we sat and watched our old memories and our just-created ones burning right before our eyes. By the time the fire was finally contained (the smoke continued long into the next morning), the wee hours of the morning were approaching. Twenty-four homes were gutted, and countless families were changed forever that night.

My parents took us to their home to settle in for a few hours of sleep. Suddenly I was a little kid again needing my parents' protection. Jim remained strong, as men will in times of crisis. I cried myself to sleep in Jim's arms, under the safety of my parents' roof. If I thought the toughest part was over, I was dead wrong. In a few hours, reality would set in. We would start to pick through the ashes, searching for our lives under the soot.

Mid-morning, the next day, we met at a local diner, before heading for the first look at our apartment. Relatives from both sides of our family and friends gathered together for breakfast and to form a game plan. Some relatives traveled from as far as seventy-five miles away. Quickly, the group divided into small working teams. One group headed to K-mart and Hills for clothes, toiletries (we didn't even own a toothbrush!), and supplies for digging through the ashes. Another group headed to the grocery store for food and drinks to keep the workers going. A final group was in charge of searching the apartment.

Jim and I were part of the group that went straight to the apartment. We arrived at exactly 11:00 A.M., the time we were told we could go inside. There was lots of confusion and chaos. The fire marshal needed to authorize people to go inside, and we had to sign releases. We were told, "You have five minutes to get all the stuff you can. You may or may not be let back in again." Those words still ring in my mind. How was I even going to walk in the door, much less get everything that mattered, in five minutes?

Jim and his brother entered first. Jim is a structural engineer by profession. He wanted to check out the stability and safety of the building before I went in. To this day, I think he went in first because he needed to come to terms with it first and then help prepare me.

The fire marshal changed his mind and said we could search the rest of the day. What a relief to not be forced to do this gruesome task in five minutes or less. My first walk into the apartment was the most difficult. I had never been into a burned building before, and I will never forget the smell and sight. Smoke, dust, soot, and water covered everything in what once was our apartment. Most things were undistinguishable. As family came back from their rounds and filtered into the apartment, they encouraged us to let the demolishing crew just gut it. Jim was certain that if we looked, we would find remnants of our past. Thanks to Jim's perseverance and meticulous searching, many of our treasured items were salvaged.

We stayed at a Red Cross–sponsored hotel that night. Family and friends both offered us housing, but we needed some personal space. We needed time to grieve our old home and begin to make plans for our future. Where would we live? What should we do next?

The next day, the long and tedious work started. Armed with shovels, picks, metal detectors, and gloves, we started the painstaking search for our life buried under the soot. While most of the other apartment dwellers signed off for demolition, we continued to search day after day. We searched for seven straight days and nights—often twelve or more hours at a time. We both took two weeks off of work to get our lives back together. Many of our family and friends came day after day to help. Our employers were very compassionate and generous, too. In fact, Jim's employer matched dollar for dollar the contributions of the employees to our fire fund.

A few days after the fire, the property management company moved us to a townhouse building a block away in the complex. Each night, as we finished our search, we returned to our temporary home. Our first night, we had one just-bought mattress, a cardboard table, two folding chairs, paper products, and a few pieces of clothing to fill a two-bedroom townhouse. Often it was late in the evening until we'd return from the site, but we were always surprised to see dinner waiting, new and used items sitting on our patio or porch stoop, and monetary gifts in the mailbox.

Many of the gifts were from family and friends, but some were also from strangers. One stranger sent us money to buy our mothers flowers and cards for Mother's Day. We know it was a stranger who shared this gift of kindness, as family and friends knew that Jim's mother passed away years before.

As we spent days searching, we started to piece our life back together. Miraculously, my wedding gown had survived untouched. The box was completely charred, but the dress didn't have a mark. A piece of drywall had fallen over the dress and protected it. We lost our wedding album, but the photographer had the negatives and gave them to us for free. As the days turned into weeks, and the gifts and money kept pouring in, we started to feel a little like the Baileys in *It's a Wonderful Life*. Friends whom we hadn't seen or talked to in years sent us gifts. Some friends even repurchased the gifts they had given us as wedding presents.

Thanks to the generous and giving nature of so many, that same summer we were able to build our first home. On our own savings, it would have certainly taken us another two to three years. Family and friends joined together to help build our house and make it a home. Our home, which we still happily occupy today, is much more than walls, floors, and ceilings. It is our special haven that grew from the love and friendship of a small-town community. We feel blessed every day.

Some may say (and have said), "It seems like you two really have your share of bad luck." Actually, we feel quite the opposite. We couldn't ask for a better life, especially since we share it together. Roommates for life!

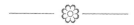

Ronda and Jim Stump live in Elizabethtown, Pennsylvania. They still live in the home they built after the fire. They are the proud and devoted parents of two adorable, fun-loving, and spirited children, Abigail and Allyson. They continue to be supported by a strong network of family and friends and remain each other's best friends. Ronda says, "It's a wonderful life!"

The First True Love of My Life

Tammy Harrison

*A*t the age of fifteen, I was told by a counselor that I had no emotions. I didn't feel a thing. It was very true, though I didn't realize it at the time. He told me that I really only had one choice to have a fulfilling life—learn to love.

Tragically, when I was eleven, our dad died of a cerebral hemorrhage caused by an aneurysm at the base of his brain. Suddenly, as the oldest boy, my brother Mike had to fill some large shoes. He was only thirteen. I remember bits and pieces of our childhood, and Mike was not usually part of those memories. He kept to himself and didn't play with me or my two younger brothers. He could usually be found parked in front of the television or working on some scrap heap of a motorcycle in the barn.

After Dad died, Mom was unable to cope. We lived on welfare in a trailer house we borrowed from an aunt. Mom had never had to earn a living for our family, let alone take care of five children all by herself. She turned to alcohol and drugs for comfort and to escape from her life.

Shortly after Dad died, I found Mom smiling one day. She had received the life insurance check. We had no idea what that meant, but the very next day we had a new car and Mom started disappearing more often, leaving us to care for ourselves. Our older sister became our primary caregiver while Mom drank herself into oblivion. We literally carried her to bed each night.

A few weeks after receiving the money, Mom left, and she never came back. My brothers were sent to live with my dad's oldest brother in Missouri. My sister moved in with relatives in our hometown in Iowa. I was the middle, obnoxious, mind-of-her-own girl who looked like my mother (shameful to my father's family), and I was not wanted. I became a ward of the state and was sent to live with some family friends.

My mother killed herself shortly afterward, but I felt nothing. I couldn't even cry at her funeral.

By this time, I had lived in two bad foster homes and had been invited to leave my hometown and move in with an aunt and uncle. I did not know how to be a part of a family, and I didn't know how to love or how to accept love. Chuck and Lynn gave me guidance, supported me through my completion of high school with honors, and reinforced the morals and values that I had learned as a child. They were like the stick that a tightrope walker holds. I could count on them, even if I had done wrong, to discuss the situation, mete out proper punishment, and move forward. They attended my high school extracurricular activities and made me a part of their family.

Even still, I remained too shut down to really know what love felt like.

Throughout the six years of being away from my family, I tried desperately to keep in contact with my brothers. Boys will be boys, and they were not much for writing letters. I lived in Nebraska and they in Missouri, with relatives from different sides of a feuding family. We never had a chance to get together.

After two years of college, I made up my mind to leave school, and I left Nebraska. I tried the army and moved in with some friends until I graduated from cosmetology school in Iowa. All the while, I knew that I needed to reestablish a relationship with my brothers. We needed the chance to be siblings without the extended family's intervention.

I moved to Missouri, and it was then that my oldest brother Mike and I started planting the seeds that would grow into the first real love of my life. I didn't even know if I was capable of loving, but I knew I had to try. I already knew what life would be like without feeling love. Mike had married and was living the same way he had in our youth—with not much motivation to do anything when he wasn't working but a lot of desire to make things better for him and his wife, Vickie. I started spending Sundays with Mike and Vickie. We laughed and cried and shared ourselves with each other in ways we had never been allowed to throughout the years.

Sundays started turning into entire weekends, and our lives became intertwined. I came to realize that this was what a family was—being a part of something without effort and with the comfort of unconditional love and respect.

Mike opened up my heart. Up until I shared love with Mike, I did not cry and I did not allow others to place their problems on me. I had no compassion, no feelings, nothing. Once I got a feel for the true meaning of love, I exploded! I laughed and I cried and I was alive. Thanks to Mike, I was living life.

My brother Mike may have been my first true love, but because of him, I opened up to the second great love of my life—my husband, John. I met John, a doctoral student at the University of Missouri, when he frequented the bar where I worked. We hit it off immediately and began spending time together and with Mike and Vickie. Mike gave his approval of John, and I proposed to him.

Mike cried when I got married, and he cried when my husband accepted a new job at a university in Texas and we moved. I cried, too, for many days and nights. The one person I cared about, outside of my husband, was miles and states away. John held me until the hurt subsided and reminded me that "love never ends, it just grows and grows no matter how far apart you are."

Mike and I talked to each other on the telephone at least once a week, and we met for long weekends together at a halfway point between our homes. Mike and Vickie didn't have children, so I shared the pregnancy and the birth of our first daughter with them. They were able to hold Keara just minutes after she was born, and we cried again. Even though we had been separated for so long, I could no longer imagine my life without him.

The Saturday before Father's Day in 1997, my husband and I were camping with our daughter. I was pregnant with child number two. I waited anxiously all day to call Mike, because I had just been to the doctor and heard the new baby's heartbeat for the first time. I had recorded the precious sounds so that Mike could hear them. That evening, I called and shared the joy of parenthood with one who truly should have been a father.

"Sounds like a freight train," he exclaimed with joy. I could see him smiling from ear to ear all the way through the phone lines! We caught up on our lives and said good-bye.

It was the last time I ever talked to him.

Mike died on Father's Day in 1997, of a cerebral hemorrhage caused by an aneurysm at the base of his brain. The family genetic curse had struck again. Another loved one was pulled from my life.

Mike lives on for me, for his widow, and for the rest of our family. In every family situation, in every decision I make, I take the time to ask myself, "What would Mike think of this?" I know he's grinning now as he reads this story I needed to tell. Keara, our oldest, is now six. She occasionally comes to me, saying she has been talking to Mike in her dreams. I am sure he is with us every day.

Mike gave me what no other person had been able to— the ability to experience the emotion we call love. You might be asking, "Wasn't the pain you experienced in losing

Mike so unbearable that you might have been better off numb as before?"

As much as the loss of Mike hurts every day, his presence in my life is what I choose to focus on. He's there when I hug my daughter and feel love that is beyond words. He was there when I celebrated a tenth wedding anniversary with my beloved husband this year. Without Mike, I wouldn't be a whole person, experiencing every emotion imaginable.

I can choose to focus on Mike's death, or on the life that he gave me. I wasted enough years suffering. I choose life. Mike, I know you are watching over me right now. I just want to say, "Thanks. I love you!"

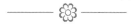

Tammy Harrison is a wife and mother of four children ages six and under, who give her the opportunity to feel love every day of her life. She is still happily married to John, an extension specialist in agricultural waste management. They live on fifty acres in a log house in northern Utah. Tammy is a home-based working mom. She specializes in marketing and creativity for small businesses and is currently the independent creative representative for Home-Based Working Moms, an association dedicated to helping bring working moms closer to their children.

Don't Feel Sorry for Me—I'm Blessed!

Theresa Blume

I was born with partial hearing in one ear, and no hearing at all in the other. People used to feel sorry for me, thinking of me as a poor little deaf girl, and others just thought I was stuck up because I wouldn't answer their questions. I felt the worst shame when people thought I was dumb because I would guess at what they said and answer the wrong thing.

To learn how to listen in other ways, I found solace in my animals, whom I learned to understand without human words. I learned how to listen to the trees when I put my cheek against their bark. When I was given a guitar I put my ear against it and fell in love with the warm sound. Since I can't understand the words to songs I hear, I started to write my own, and that way I also got the music right. Nobody could say it was wrong because it was my own song!

Because I don't hear the little distractions of life like refrigerators running or distant thunder or leaves rustling, my spiritual connection with God has been strengthened. I learned how to feel God's presence in the wind, and I can hear God's voice easily. Some people have told me I have great wisdom and want to know how to hear God. I tell them I myself am not wise, but because of my lack of physical hearing, I seem to be able to hear better spiritually.

In compensation for my hearing loss, I have an excellent sense of smell. If my children light a match downstairs or even outside, I smell it immediately. I have never used an oven timer because my nose tells me exactly when my baking is done. My nose warns me when trouble is near in the form of drugs like marijuana, especially when someone uses incense or perfume to cover up the smell. I once realized that someone I knew was doing cocaine, simply because he was breathing faster than normal, something I noticed because I have to watch people closely to hear them. When something doesn't feel right to me, my eyes usually tell me that something is wrong or different, but sometimes my nose susses out the problem first.

Another wonderful benefit of my hearing loss is when people talk, I must look at them to know what they are saying. People love being paid attention to, so it helps my relationships. The eyes really are the windows to the soul. They tell the truth no matter what the words are saying. Lip reading lets you see what people want you to know, but their eyes will tell you the truth of what they are feeling on the inside.

Being almost deaf has brought me much closer to my husband. He is a soft-spoken person, so we must be within close range of each other in order to communicate. He knows I need him when we are in public, so he listens intently and tells me what I missed. We have a special togetherness that other couples don't always create with one another.

Because I am able to hear God more clearly than people who are distracted by all the noise in their lives, I have counseled more than two thousand people. The spiritual wisdom gained from being able to hear God within my soul seems to bring others a peace that they can't find in the hearing world.

There are wonderful advantages to being able to take my hearing aides out and not hear everything the rest of the world hears, like the television blaring or people whispering behind my back or noises in the night that keep others awake (although my other senses wake me up if needed). I don't hear traffic going by my house or wild neighborhood parties or far-away barking dogs. I am not distracted by buzzing insects or worried about distant thunder. I also don't hear people wrapping presents in another room, so I am always surprised when I am given a present that my children have managed to keep secret from me!

My children find it fun to sneak up on me and spook me once in a while. Unfortunately for them, I usually smell them first and surprise them with orders to take a shower!

I pray for a lot of things, but I don't pray for better hearing. I consider it a blessing, and not a disability at all.

God tells me when my children are in trouble, whether they are next to me or a thousand miles away. My dog tells me who is not trustworthy. My kids have to look me in the face to tell me anything; they absolutely cannot lie without my knowing it because I see their eyes. My husband and I have a special relationship built on trust and support.

I do not feel like I have been cheated out of something most people have. On the contrary, I have been given something special that most people are longing for—close connections with my family, friends, and God. How blessed I am!

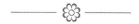

Theresa Blume is an inspirational writer known for her weekly "Blooming Inspirations" and freelance writing. She has recorded her songs on an album called *Soaring Higher* and has spoken to groups about her book *Hope for Tomorrow*. She is happily married and has three children.

I'm Just Fine!

Beth Fryer

My parents still say, "We told you so." I know they're waiting to hear me say, "You're right, I regret marrying Joe."

Twenty-five years ago, I was young, sheltered, and naive. Joe had two former wives and three children. The daughter from his second marriage was in his custody. It was among the most unlikely matches imaginable. We have since spoken of the fact that our daughter—well, *his* daughter, then—was the main reason we married. He knew she needed a mom who was more involved than her birth mother had been, and I wanted a child who was already "housebroken." My parents threw the proverbial fit, even threatening to disown me, their only daughter. When I went ahead with my plans anyway, they relented and paid for our lovely wedding.

Our marriage was difficult. Yes, of course there were good times ... but not enough of them. I knew I was the injured party, as Joe had one affair after another, while I tried to make things change. By then, his daughter was my child too, and I dreaded the thought of leaving and losing her as well, with no legal bonds to hold her to me. After five and a half years of struggling and hurting, an affair grew serious enough that Joe told me he wanted a divorce. The word had been uttered many times before, but this time we both knew our marriage was over.

Despite some angry arguments, we parted on friendly terms. He helped me move, we continued to see one another for a while, off and on, and most important, I was blessed to share joint custody of our daughter, then twelve years old. I saw her almost every day.

But the blessings didn't end there. Joe didn't marry that "other woman." He married another young woman who was kind to me as I struggled to let go of the marriage, and became a friend as we shared our daughter—*and* the schnauzer. They married when our daughter was fourteen. When she left Joe four years later, I was the friend Joe called, at 5:00 A.M. His daughter and I tried our best to see him through the difficult time.

Several months later, we decided to try again for a few more years. For most of that time, I didn't even let my parents know that he and I were seeing one another. When Mom eventually suspected and asked, I admitted that we were "dating" again, and we pretty much avoided the subject. I knew they were concerned, but they joined the ranks of my friends, all hoping I'd survive this experiment without getting hurt again.

We didn't make it. Fast-forward to today, five years later. My parents and some friends still think of my relationship with Joe as my life's greatest disaster, but the blessings from my life with him far outweigh the bad times. In those last few years when we tried to make it work, we had a lovely, comfortable relationship and were able to enjoy our daughter's wedding together, as well as many holidays and other happy times with her. We had the chance to talk about the years we were married, and come to terms with the ways we had hurt each other. Yes, even that—for I came to know I wasn't blameless. And we apologized. The wounds healed, and our friendship grew. We parted again, this time we knew for good, but without anger, as friends.

I am grateful for the years I spent with Joe, and happy with who I am now as a single woman. I have no regrets about the years spent with him, just gratitude. My life is surely richer because he was part of it.

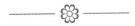

Beth Fryer is a sixth-grade teacher in Lebanon, Pennsylvania. She enjoys spending time with her family—her daughter and son-in-law, three grandchildren, and her parents. Her other passions are her dachshund, her cats, reading, and experiencing spirituality, gratitude, and life's wonderful divine order.

Enough Stuff!

Tracy Callow

My parents split up when I was sixteen, and thus began a steady diet of frequent moves, which took me from my home state of Texas to Maryland. I was in a hurry to be independently established as an adult (which I thought of as having my own stuff). As soon as I graduated high school, I started college, where I met my husband, Chris, and we happily tied the knot a bit over a year later.

My husband and I were determined to live the American dream as soon as possible. For us, that meant a house near water, a boat, two cars, pets, two children, domestic and exotic travel, an impressive organic landscape, and enough financial freedom to hunt for and collect antiques as we desired. After several years of marriage, and two successful careers, my husband and I bought our first house on an island in the Chesapeake Bay of Maryland. It was exactly what we wanted as we looked forward to beginning a family. But then our American dream took a bit of a detour.

After enjoying our new house for two years, my husband and I were both laid off from our jobs within one month of each other. We combined our talents (mine as a graphic designer and his as a computer and network technician) and started a business aimed at supplying and maintaining computer equipment and designing logos, brochures, and Web sites for local businesses.

Anyone who has ever launched a business on a shoestring can predict what happened next. Soon our mortgage payment was late for the first time. By the time we had the funds for one mortgage payment, the mortgage lender wouldn't accept anything less than two months' payments, plus exorbitant late fees. So it steamrolled, and we were always a month behind, but they wouldn't accept our partial payment. After countless letters and phone calls to the lender over the course of two more years, it was determined that the only way they would work with us on a repayment plan would be for us to file full bankruptcy. We hesitated but decided to go through with it, since it was the only way to save the house.

Since we were going to stay in the house, we figured we could ride out seven years of bad credit with no problem. After more than seven years of marriage, I found out I was pregnant with our first child. We were both elated. It seemed like perfect timing, since we were finally over the battle of saving our house. We had a thriving business in our small community, and I was set to work from home once our little one arrived.

A month later, when I was nearly three months pregnant, our biggest crisis yet came in the mail. Our county courthouse sent us a letter saying that we had one week to vacate the house, as they were auctioning it on the courthouse steps, a few steps away from some of our major clients.

It turned out that our loan had been sold to a new lender who made no deals regarding late payments. It was not a good week, to say the least. A couple of days before we moved, the creditor from whom we leased our truck appropriated it during the night one month before payoff. They didn't tolerate bankruptcy, despite our impeccable payment history.

The whole ordeal was humiliating, especially since we were young, well-known business owners in a small old-school community and active in our community association. What we realized, as we moved hastily into our new rental home, in the rain, is that what we needed was a lot less stuff!

For several reasons, embarrassment included, we decided to get a fresh start and relocate. My husband secured a job in Austin, Texas, and we started packing. I planned to hold on to many of my clients, since most of my work was done through FedEx and the Internet anyway. Just before moving with our new daughter to Texas, we had a yard sale to end all yard sales and made several hundred dollars. It was liberating!

We trekked across the country, and once we arrived in Texas, met up with another fiasco. The moving company held our goods for five weeks (even the beds!), then promptly lost several key items—client records included. After struggling to regain our stuff from the movers, we had yet another yard sale and donated even more. It was even easier this time. I couldn't wait to shed myself of as much stuff as we could part with. If we had achieved the American dream as we imagined, we would have been miserable. We began attending church regularly and found much more satisfaction there than in our previous expeditions to flea markets and antique sales. We are no longer living with such a heavy weight of responsibility on our shoulders, and we feel more spontaneous with our time. We are having a lot more fun, and one other side benefit of streamlining our lives is that the house sure is easier to clean!

Getting rid of stuff now makes us happier than acquiring it! We have created a new American dream—simple living.

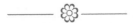

Tracy Callow is a part-time graphic designer and work-from-home mom. Tracy, her husband, Chris, their daughter, Gabrielle, two dogs, and one cat currently live in Beaufort, South Carolina, but plan to be living back in Texas by publication of this book. She is currently writing a book on living an uncluttered life.

Walking Till the Day I Die

Vicki Herrity

*M*y granddad used to work for the electricity company in Belfast, Northern Ireland, putting up the telegraph poles that hold the electricity wires. On one particular day, in January of 1969, he was up a forty-foot pole, and in those days they didn't have the vehicle with the crane and box to hoist the workmen up, so they had to climb the pole.

He had put up quite a few poles, but on this day he let his attention wander and he slipped. In the split second that it took to realize he was going to land headfirst, he managed to twist himself around and land on his feet. However, because of the distance, the landing caused him to shatter every bone in his feet and his legs right up to his knees. A passing priest witnessed what had happened and gave him the last rites there and then even though he wasn't Catholic.

The doctors told him that he would never walk again. He spent the next eighteen months crawling about in his family home, confined to the kitchen and living room. A bucket was used to help him with his bathroom needs, since they had an outside toilet and he slept on the sofa at night. During that time, my mum, his daughter, got married. He couldn't walk her down the aisle. He realized that unless he did something about it, he would miss out on many more occasions.

For the next twelve months he worked on building up the strength in his legs. His whole family helped in holding him while he tried to stand for the first time. This was the hardest part because his legs were like Jell-O.

Some days were better than others, but he kept at it until he could stand sixty seconds by himself before his legs gave in. You can imagine the determination and persistence he must have had to keep on going and to keep trying until he eventually could walk by himself. It took him a total of fifty weeks before he was finally able to walk for hours a day, unattended.

My granddad was so grateful for having the use of his legs back that he made a promise to spend an hour each day out walking. For every day of his life after that, he did just that. He had a motorbike license, but he never rode the bike again. He walked everywhere. If he needed to go a distance, he would get the bus. I can always remember him with a walking stick, but he didn't need it. He said it was for protection from dogs and possibly the opportunist mugger.

Granddad lived until the grand old age of eighty-three, when stomach cancer took him from us. Up until then, he was a very independent man. My mum used to joke that he needed a secretary; she had to make an appointment to see him because he was out so often. He made so many friends on his travels. He made time every day to go visit "the old people." Many of these people were ten to twenty years younger than him, but they looked forward to his visits because they were confined to their homes.

Granddad's accident actually improved both the quality and longevity of his life. His constant walking kept him healthy and strong and enabled him to befriend people whom he wouldn't have met otherwise. The vendor at the fish market told us that he knew that Granddad was gone before he actually heard the official news. Why? Because Granddad visited every Tuesday; he never missed it. When Granddad didn't show up to visit his old friend at the fish market that Tuesday, the vendor knew he had to be dead. That was the only thing that would have kept granddad away from his regular visits.

Granddad was a man greatly admired by his family, even today. His father died when Granddad was nineteen, and being the eldest of twelve children, he helped raise his eleven siblings. He brought in his share of money with his mother to keep everyone clothed and fed. His wife, Elizabeth, said they would have married sooner only he was so intent on looking after the family. They didn't marry until they were thirty, when everyone was old enough to work and look after themselves. He reassured her by saying they would grow old together, but when she was sixty-four, he retired early to look after her when she was diagnosed with cancer, which eventually claimed her life.

Granddad didn't think of himself as a religious man, even though he did believe in God. During his last few days he had a local minister visit him who reassured him that he had a place in heaven. There was never a doubt in anyone's mind who knew Granddad. His well-attended funeral was a testimony to how many people's lives he touched. His shattered legs had turned my granddad into a healer of hearts.

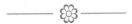

Vicki Herrity is the granddaughter of Thomas Beattie. She has inherited only a fraction of her granddad's determination and persistence, but it did cause her to prove her high school teachers wrong when they said she wouldn't get high enough grades to go to university. She went on to start her own business at age twenty-five. Her message to anyone reading the above story is that if a fifty-eight-year-old man could learn to walk again, then think what you can achieve. There is nothing holding you back. Start today, and do it. Achieve your dreams!

Acknowledgments

Every author thanks her editor and says something like, "Without my editor, this book never would have happened." Well, I'm no exception! I take credit for collecting and editing these stories, but the idea for this book originated with my superb editor, Paula Munier, who after dreaming up the concept asked me to do the project for her. Paula, you were inspired. I'm so glad you thought of me. This was the perfect book for me, and you knew it all along.

Thanks to all the authors who submitted their stories for consideration, both those who were selected as finalists and those who were not. It takes great courage to submit a true story about a personal experience, knowing that only a small percentage of applicants will make it to the final cut. Those of you who didn't make it in, I want you to know that I was touched by your stories and I know that they will find the right home. And to those authors who made it to the final stage, every one of you is a poster child for the "half-full" attitude.

Stephen, my husband and life partner, I am so grateful that both you and I live by this philosophy. When faced with one of many challenges in our marriage, we have consistently chosen the path of optimism and hope. Marrying you was the best decision I've ever made.

Hashem, you are the reason why I live by the statement "Gam Zu Letovah"—"this too is for the best." I believe that there is a divine plan for my life and that whatever happens is ultimately for the best. I feel your presence in my life, and I am grateful.

Finally, thank you to the competent staff at Fair Winds who took the stories via email and turned them into something pretty on the printed page.

Contact Information

Allen, Mary Emma
I Never Knew Who I Would Be
Plymouth, NH
fax: 603-536-4851
email: *me.allen@juno.com,*
jetent@cyberportal.net
Web site:
www.homepage.fcgnetwo

Asenjo, Bill, Ph.D., C.R.C.
From Bars to Books
email: *basenjo@avalon.net*

Blume, Theresa
Don't Feel Sorry for Me—
I'm Blessed!
email: *theresa@tznet.com*

Buechel, Darlene A.
Baking Up a Storm
N5204 McHugh Rd.
Chilton, WI 53014
phone: 920-849-9406

Callow, Tracy
Enough Stuff!
6116 Jeff Loop
San Antonio, TX 78238
email: *gistudio@islc.net*

Casey, Rayelenn Sparks
Eleven-Plus
429 Camp Meeting Rd.
Landisville, PA 17538
phone: 717-892-3080
email: *Rayelenn@aol.com*

Douglas, Freda
Lavender Walls
2442 Azalea Ln.
Wauchula, FL 33873
phone: 863-773-5764
email: *cxzfd@strato.net*

Friedman, Sally
Monkey Bars
phone: 856-235-1272
email: *pinegander@aol.com*

Frost, Penny
No More Fear
phone: 207-783-1998
email: *penrich@megalink.net*

Fryer, Beth
I'm Just Fine!
320 E. Lehman St.
Lebanon, PA 17046
email: *bfryer@nbn.net*

Gibbs, Nancy B.
A God-Given Confidence
P.O. Box 53
Cordele, GA 31010
email: *Daiseydood@aol.com*

Gross, Jeff
Getting Fired Got Me Fired Up
email: *Jgross9258@aol.com*

Haggerty, Deb, M.B.A., C.M.C.
No Longer the Ugly Stepmother
9725 Blandford Rd.
Orlando, FL 32827-7039
phone: 407-856-2897;
1-888-332-7757
email: *Deb@DebHaggerty.com*
Web site:
www.DebHaggerty.com

Hammack, Barbara
I'm Still Standing!
3806 Archer Pl.
Kensington, MD 20895
phone: 301-942-8153

Harrison, Tammy
The First True Love of My Life
email: *tammyh@jdharrison.com*

Hays, Roland
Amazing Hands
9238 E. Palm Tree Dr.
Scottsdale, AZ 85255-5544
phone: 480-502-8870
email: *rolandhays@aol.com*

Herrity, Vicki
Walking Till the Day I Die
email: *vicki@netplosion.com*

Holtz-Oxley, Lorrell
Johnny
email:
johnsbuddies@comcast.net
Web site:
*www.mywebpages.comcast.net/
johnsbuddies*

Jaffe, Azriela
Sweet Sarah
793 Sumter Dr.
Yardley, PA 19067

email: *azriela@mindspring.com*
Web site: *www.azriela.com*

Kasdin, Karin
Emmy and Sara
email: *KKasdin@aol.com*

Kiser, Roger
I'm a Good Girl
100 Northridge Dr.
Brunswick, GA 31525
email:
trampolineone@webtv.net
Web site: *www.geocities.com/
thesadorphanfoundation*

Kittle, Risë A.
Serendipity
1403 Rocky Creek Rd.
Harrison, GA 31035
phone: 478-240-0604
email: *cocobabe@dfnow.com*

Ledue, Gene
Standing Up for Downhill
31 Keswick Rd.
South Portland, ME 04106
email:
eledue@unumprovident.com

Maddox, Latoya Chivon
It Doesn't Keep Me from Smiling
2600 Belmont Ave.
Inglis House

Philadelphia PA 19131
Meyer, Carol A.
I Am the One
email:
CarolAMeyer@SoftHome.net

Mooney, Patty
Heightened Senses
email:
Patty@newuniquevideos.com
Web site:
www.Crystalpyramid.com

Oliver, Jennifer
Walking Trellis
email: *four_ears@msn.com*

Ryan, Robin
Quest for Fame
14404 SE 93rd St.
Newcastle, WA 98059
phone: 425-226-0414
Web site: *www.RobinRyan.com*

Russell, Cheryl
Home, Sweet Home
email: *crussell@mwt.net*

Sander, Jennifer Basye
Another Miracle, Not My Own
P.O. Box 2463
Granite Bay, CA 95746

Sefton, Jaime Strauss
Interrupted Love
P.O. Box 7782
Gold Cast Mail Centre
Surfers/Bundall, Qld 4217,
Australia

Shineberg, Liesel
Fried-Egg Sandwiches
Liesel Shineberg
320 P St.
Rock Springs, WY 82901
email: *liesel@allwest.net*

Silverman, Robin L.
The $4,000,000 Question
Robin L. Silverman
email: *creativisions@yahoo.com*
Web site:
www.robinsilverman.com

Simmons, Deborah Dee
"An Answered Prayer"
1432 W. Main St.
Ionia, MI 48846
phone: 616-527-3049
email:
jdsimmons@chartermi.net,
dsimmons@ionia.k12.mi.us

Stroupe, Nanci
Lost in a Big City
123 Tide Mill Ln.
Hampton, VA 23666

phone: 757-825-8080
email: *Onenoni@aol.com*

Stump, Ronda Graby
All Was Not Lost, and Even
More Was Found
Ronda Stump
30 Woodview Dr.
Elizabethtown, PA 17022
email: *jrstump@supernet.com*

Victor, Roberta
My Cup Runneth Over
Lightbearer Presentations
email:
lightbearer@lightbearerpres.com
Web site:
www.lightbearerpres.com

Weinreich, Roiza
It Will Be Good
625 Avenue L
Brooklyn, NY 11230
phone: 718-338-4181
email: *Rdwhom@aol.com*
Web site: *www.Artscroll.com*

Wooldridge, Connie Feste
The Last Kiss
2905 Colt Dr.
Lawrence, KS 66049
phone: 785-749-0848

About the Author

Azriela Jaffe is the author of twelve books, including:

Create Your Own Luck: Eight Principles of Attracting Good Fortune Into Your Life, Love, and Work (Adams Media, 2000)

Heartwarmers, Heartwarmers of Love, and *Heartwarmers of Spirit* (Adams Media 2000, 2001, 2002)

Permission to Prosper: What Working Wives Crave from Their Husbands and How to Get It! (Prima, 2002)

Let's Go Into Business Together: Eight Secrets to Successful Business Partnering (Career Press, 2000)

Two Jews Can Still be a Mixed Marriage: Reconciling Differences Regarding Judaism in Your Marriage (New Page, 2000)

Starting from No: 10 Strategies to Overcome Your Fear of Rejection and Succeed in Business (Dearborn, 1999)

Honey, I Want to Start my Own Business: A Planning Guide for Couples (HarperBusiness, 1996)

To subscribe to her free weekly email newsletter, *Create Your Own Luck*, email azriela@mindspring.com, or visit her Web site at www.azriela.com or www.CreateYourOwnLuck.com.

If you have a "Half Full" story to share, email it to the author at azriela@mindspring.com. We will consider your story for future editions of *Half Full*.